HIGHS, LOWS, AND PLATEAUS

A path to recovery from stroke

ANNE BURLEIGH JACOBS, PT, PhD

ILLUSTRATIONS BY: STEPHEN ADAMS

authorHOUSE®

AuthorHouse™
1663 Liberty Drive
Bloomington, IN 47403
www.authorhouse.com
Phone: 1-800-839-8640

Published by AuthorHouse 3/11/2014
ISBN: 978-1-4918-6231-5 (sc)
ISBN: 978-1-4918-6230-8 (hc)
ISBN: 978-1-4918-6229-2 (e)

Library of Congress Control Number: 2014902856

CONTENTS

ACKNOWLEDGEMENTS

I want to thank my husband, Ron Jacobs, PhD and my daughters, Heather and Merel, for their insistence that I write this book and for their creative insights for the cover design. Also, thank you to Rosalie and Stephen at AuthorHouse for their assistance in creating the illustrations. Lastly, I want to acknowledge the many, many survivors of brain injury that I have been blessed to know over the years. They have shared with me the power behind personal resilience and taught me that to survive is not enough. One must also thrive.

INTRODUCTION TO THE AUTHOR

This book is inspired by years of research, teaching, and clinical practice developed around the concept of Neuroplasticity and the phenomenal capacity of the human brain and spirit to overcome injury.

The author, Anne Burleigh Jacobs PT, PhD, graduated with a Bachelors Degree in Physical Therapy in 1985 and a Doctorate in Neuroscience and Physiology in 1995. As a licensed Physical Therapist, she has worked in private hospitals, university hospitals, nursing homes, home-care settings and in her own private clinic. During graduate school she had many amazing opportunities. While at the R.S. Dow Neurological Sciences Institute in Portland Oregon, she was exposed to rat spinal cord preparations, single cell thalamic recordings in raccoons, spinal cat locomotor studies, and human balance studies. In addition to her own research under Fay Horak, PT, PhD at the R.S. Dow Neurological Sciences Institute, Dr. Jacobs was also able to study at multiple laboratories including the Biomechanics Laboratory in Waterloo, Canada; Queens Square Neurology Hospital in London, England; and Clinical Wintersol in Tenerife, Spain.

After earning her PhD, Dr. Jacobs taught neurology, neuroanatomy and human physiology at the Hogeschool Enschede in The Netherlands and was a visiting lecturer at multiple other Physical Therapy programs in The Netherlands. She also had the opportunity to assist in developing a public program and research line for Parkinson's Disease studies and assisted in graduate student projects at the University of Twente. While living in the Netherlands, Dr. Jacobs edited and contributed to the 1st edition of the textbook, NeuroScience: Fundamentals for Rehabilitation.

Upon returning to the United States, Dr. Jacobs began teaching continuing education courses through The Dogwood Institute and became one of the founders of the Peninsula Stroke Association (now Pacific Stroke Association) where she served as the Executive Director during the first three years of the fledgling non-profit organization. She developed all of the programs and has spoken with hundreds of small groups to teach about the warning signs of stroke and the potential of post-stroke rehabilitation.

Pursuing her love of teaching, Dr. Jacobs sought out opportunities as an instructor at numerous universities in degree programs for physical therapy as well as at continuing education courses for health care professionals. At the same time, building her private practice – SensoMotor Neurological Rehabilitation, LLC. Recently, she has provided consultation to companies developing robotics, bionics, and orthotics for neurological rehabilitation.

It is with this diverse background and an ever-burgeoning love of neuroscience, that Dr. Jacobs writes this book. It is an attempt to bridge the gap between medicine, rehabilitation, basic science research and the stroke survivor. A friend in graduate school once dubbed her as "The Librarian", because of her voracious appetite for reading research and neuroscience text books in her spare time and then knowing which reference to bring into a conversation at any give time. The goal of this book is to bridge the gap by creating a useful and easily understandable connection for the reader.

Recovery from neurological injury is a long, long road with highs, lows, and plateaus – but each day is a new day toward reaching one's goal.

PREFACE

As a new graduate from physical therapy school, I took my first job at a small private hospital in Denver, Colorado. A new physiatrist – doctor of physical medicine and rehabilitation - had recently joined the staff and he was going to develop a comprehensive stroke rehabilitation program with PT, OT, Speech and Family services. I was so excited to be part of something that fueled my fascination with the brain and nervous system!

I still remember the day I met Steve. Well, I can't say that we met, but at least I knew about him. He was a young man and he was in the Neuro ICU. I was working with a patient on the other side of the curtain, when I overheard the neurosurgeon tell Steve's wife that she should accept the fact that her husband would need to go to a care facility/ nursing home. With the severity of the stroke he suffered, he would never walk again or be able to live independently.

I was bold. I was brazen. I was naïve. I approached the neurosurgeon and told him about the new comprehensive stroke rehabilitation program and suggested that he refer Steve for physical therapy. He actually laughed and then said, "O.K. Good luck with this one". Anyone who knows me knows that I love a challenge. But it was more than that. I truly believe in the potential of the human brain and the resilience of the human spirit. I believed that a young man with a new wife, a new career and a chance at life would make a good recovery.

There were other therapists who worked with Steve, but I remember Pam. She and I put in a lot of extra time together. Too much time has passed for me to remember all of the details of in-patient, out-patient, etc... but I do remember that there was a "Talent Show". We were showcasing the progress that people had made in therapy and Steve was in the talent show. We sent an invitation to the neurosurgeon and he came to the show. I will never forget seeing Steve walk on to the stage. He limped. It was the typical stroke pattern of walking, but he was walking and he was wearing a magician's hat. He boldly asked the audience for a volunteer to assist with his magic trick and then he chose the one person who did not volunteer... The surgeon joined Steve on the stage and inspected the empty magician's hat from which Steve later pulled a rabbit. Then they shook hands.

Two years later, I had moved to Seattle, Washington when I received a letter that had been forwarded from the hospital in Denver. It was a thank you note from Steve. He had a new baby and was working again as an architect, and he just wanted to say thank you.

For the past 28 years, I have lived and taught the principles of Neuroplasticity. By using my skills as a therapist, my love of teaching, and my understanding of fundamental neuroscience research I have tried to bridge the gap between clinical practice and research.

The brain is amazing and the strength and resilience of the human psyche is equally as amazing. In the following pages, I hope to provide a framework for understanding the stages and process of recovery to inspire stroke survivors and their families to move along the path of recovery. It is important to recognize that "recovery" does not always mean being 100% restored to the pre-injury condition. Recovery is a process and each individual sets their own goals and determines their own acceptable outcome. It is important to set reachable goals and once those are achieved set new goals. Surround yourself with positive people who believe in you. Remember that just because someone else tells you that you *cannot* do something does not mean it is true.

While this book focuses on recovery from stroke, I do want to emphasize that much of the information applies to recovery from any traumatic injury to the nervous system including traumatic brain injury and spinal cord injury. There will be highs, lows and plateaus. It is a long path, but the resilience of the human spirit never ceases to amaze me.

CHAPTER ONE

WHAT IS A STROKE?

This book focuses on the mechanisms of recovery from a stroke, but to understand recovery one needs a basic understanding of injury. Much of the information applies to other injuries of the central nervous system, including traumatic brain injury and spinal cord injury. In general, injury to the central nervous system involves a disruption of blood flow, inflammation, and damage to the cellular structure.

Stroke is the result of disrupted blood flow to the brain. The more technical term is *Cerebral Vascular Accident (CVA)*: cerebral = brain, vascular = blood flow, accident = unexpected. The more attention-catching media term is *Brain Attack* – much like a Heart Attack. A heart attack occurs when blood flow to the heart is interrupted and the cells that are electrical in nature stop functioning. Likewise, a brain attack occurs when the blood flow to the brain is interrupted causing the cells that are electrical in nature to stop communicating. The symptoms of the brain attack (stroke) will depend on which pathway for blood flow is interrupted and thus the corresponding region of cells whose communication is compromised.

There are two main types of stroke:

Ischemic and *Hemorrhagic.*

With the <u>*ischemic*</u> stroke, there is actually a blockage in the blood vessel preventing the flow of blood past that point. A clot that forms in place (thrombosis) or a clot that has broken loose and traveled from some distant blood vessel (embolism) forms a blockage. Cells on the far side of the blockage are denied blood flow and begin to die.

With the <u>*hemorrhagic*</u> stroke, there is actually a bleeding vessel within the brain environment. The most common hemorrhagic causes include an Aneurysm, an Arterio-Venous Malformation, and a Hematoma following a blow to the head. Blood is actually toxic to neurons (brain cells). Usually, neurons never come into direct contact with blood. Instead, a small helper cell called an astrocyte places one foot on a blood vessel and one foot on a brain cell and then oxygen and nutrition diffuse out of the blood vessel, through the astrocyte and to the brain cell. So, when there is a bleed in the brain environment, cells in direct contact with blood begin to die.

As neurons die, the cell walls collapse and the chemical content of the cell is released, poisoning other cells in the surrounding area. But, it is important to appreciate that not all of the cells in the area die. Brain cells are pretty clever. Recognizing that the brain environment has become a war zone, the surviving cells turn down their energy production and go silent...waiting for the danger to pass.

That war zone is a mess – a zone of swelling,
cellular debris, and chemical toxins.

Last winter, there was a terrible storm that moved through the mountains where we live. Trees were down everywhere and with them were downed power lines and phone lines. No Power, No Communication. Silence after the storm.

Neurons are electrical cells. They conduct a signal and communicate with other cells via a chemical-electrical cascade. When neurons die or go silent, they simply stop communicating. The goal of recovery is to either repair the downed lines of communication or build new lines of communication so that cells are able to receive and send messages again. Sometimes this happens quite quickly - almost spontaneously - sometimes it takes a long time and a lot of work, and sometimes, the barriers to recovery are just too great. It is very difficult to know which survivors will continue to recover and which have reached their limit. Individual determination, finances, the survivor's pre-stroke health, personality and environment are important components in their recovery.

~ Sometimes recovery means regaining past abilities and sometimes it means learning new ways. ~

NOTES:

CHAPTER TWO

EMERGENCY TREATMENT OF STROKE

I graduated with my bachelors' degree in Physical Therapy in 1985. At that time, there was not a lot that could be done in regards to the emergency treatment of stroke. By the time I earned my doctoral degree in Neuroscience and Physiology in 1995 progress was in the making. In February 1996, a clot-busting medication was approved, by the Federal Drug Administration, for the emergency treatment of stroke. This medication, tissue plasminogen activator (tPA) is able to dissolve a clot allowing blood flow to be restored to the brain, but it must be administered within only a few hours from the onset of the ischemic stroke. It doesn't work for treatment of hemorrhagic stroke. Remember, that type of stroke involves a ruptured blood vessel, not a clot or blockage. But, the introduction of tPA for emergency treatment of stroke opened the door to many recent advances in the treatment of stroke.

Advances in imaging and drug delivery have helped to lengthen the treatment window for using tPA. Clot-retrieval devices that mechanically reach into a blood vessel to remove the clot have recently come onto the treatment scene and have lengthened the treatment time window. Surgical advances have also been made in the treatment of hemorrhagic stroke.

In 2003, the Joint Commission, a nonprofit organization that accredits and certifies healthcare organizations, joined forces with the American Heart Association and American Stroke Association (AHA/ASA) to begin certification of Primary Stroke Centers (http://www. strokeassociation.org). These centers are certified to provide for emergency treatment of stroke. More than 900 hospitals nationwide have been certified. It may be worth knowing which hospitals in your area are certified.

In 2012 this accreditation process was expanded and the Joint Commission together with AHA/ASA began certification of comprehensive stroke centers. These centers are even more specialized having advanced treatment and surgical tools for the emergency management of stroke. Also, they have a team of rehabilitation professionals who specialize in treating patients following complicated strokes.

Recently, Telemedicine has been an exciting advancement in emergency treatment of stroke. This allows hospitals in even the most remote regions to have immediate access to top-notch, specialized neurologists who can guide the treatment protocol using tPA.

Eleven years ago, I knew a woman who had a stroke while enjoying a day boating on a lake in the Sierra Nevada Foothills. By the time she was transported to the local hospital and then transferred to a Primary Stroke Center that was three hours away, too much time had passed. The treatment window was closed and nothing could be done except to wait and see how bad the effects of the stroke were and then plan for rehabilitation. This year, that same small hospital in the Sierras is geared-up for telemedicine, which now may allow them to successfully treat that patient who years ago they could not.

Unfortunately, a low percentage of people having an ischemic stroke (due to clot) get to the hospital within the treatment window for using tPA. Community education is key to getting people to recognize the signs and symptoms of stroke and having enough confidence to act quickly. Community education about the warning signs as well as the risk factors for stroke also helps to lessen the fear that many stroke survivors live with daily – the fear that they will have another stroke.

The treatable risk factors include:

High Blood Pressure, High Cholesterol, Atrial Fibrillation, and Diabetes. Sometimes there are also injuries to the blood vessels themselves, which require medical attention.

The lifestyle-related risk factors include:

Tobacco use (smoking or chewing), Excessive alcohol consumption, and Obesity. The use of birth control pills, in addition to any of the other risk factors, also increases the risk for women.

Assuming a healthier lifestyle and working with your physician and a dietician is the first step in decreasing the risk factors associated with stroke.

The following chapter provides examples of the signs and symptoms of stroke. I encourage everyone to know these, because you may be the one to recognize someone else's stroke and seek emergency medical attention for them.

~ *Time Lost is Brain Lost* ~

AHA/ASA

STROKE
is a MEDICAL EMERGENCY

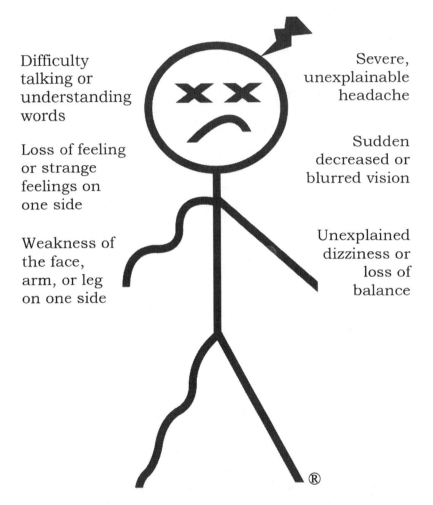

Difficulty talking or understanding words

Loss of feeling or strange feelings on one side

Weakness of the face, arm, or leg on one side

Severe, unexplainable headache

Sudden decreased or blurred vision

Unexplained dizziness or loss of balance

With two or more of these warning signs
Call 911
The first 3 hours are critical for treatment

CHAPTER THREE

STROKE STRIKES ANYWHERE, ANYTIME

It is very important for everyone to recognize the signs of stroke, because stroke strikes anywhere, anytime, across age, ethnicity, and socio-economic groups. I have never known anyone who planned on having a stroke. But, I know a lot of people who survived with minimal deficit because someone else recognized the signs and sought help. Unfortunately, in my field of work, I also know a lot of people whose symptoms of stroke went unrecognized. Remember, according to U.S. national statistics, a low percentage of stroke victims get to the hospital in time for emergency intervention.

The odd thing about a stroke is that the person having a stroke often does not fully realize that anything is wrong. When asked if they are o.k. the person having the stroke quite often says they are fine or makes up a reason to explain their behavior. Remember, it is the brain that is under attack - and this is the same brain that is supposed to be identifying that something is wrong! A brain under attack is going to have to rely on someone else to identify the problem and seek help.

The stick-figure on the preceding page is used by the Pacific Stroke Association (formerly the Peninsula Stroke Association), based in Palo Alto, California (http://www.pacificstrokeassociation.org). It was drawn by a man, Sam Frank, who had a stroke while attending a meeting. A colleague knew something was wrong and called 911. Sam was successfully treated with tPA, the clot-busting drug approved by the FDA in 1996. This simple stick-figure, represents the array of signs and symptoms of stroke. Not everyone will present with the same set of symptoms, but in general it is advised "TWO OR MORE IN COMBINATION – CALL 911"

HEADACHE – Lots of people have headaches, but this headache is often described as the "first or the worst." People report that the headache they had the day of their stroke was different than ones they had before; it was the first one like it. Also, they report it was the worst headache they had ever had. Remember, one or more of the other symptoms will accompany this headache.

CHANGE IN VISION – Any *sudden* change in vision is a warning sign that something is wrong. People will report that

- their vision grew blurry,
- they lost vision in one eye,
- a curtain fell over part of their field of sight

Sometimes stroke victims don't really lose part of their vision, but they lose the perception of vision – they can no longer decipher or understand what they see. For example, the red-octagonal sign at an intersection may appear to have some white letters or figures, but it holds no meaning. The stroke victim, may see it, but not understand that it is the familiar stop sign.

SPEECH – Any *sudden* change in the ability to speak or to comprehend language is a warning sign that something is wrong. The stroke victim may present with

- slurred speech,
- loss of speech,
- partial loss of speech with word finding problems,

OR

- they may be able to speak, but it is all nonsense.

WEAKNESS – This may present as weakness and loss of coordination of the face, hand, arm, or leg on one side of the body, OR it may be a generalized weakness and loss of coordination in both legs. Often, the stroke victim may fail to move a body part and not even be aware of it. For example, they may drag their leg when attempting to walk, be unable to lift their arm to turn off the water and instead use the other hand. They may smile or talk and not be aware that one side of the mouth is drooping.

CHANGE IN SENSATION – This symptom often accompanies the weakness or loss of coordination. People have reported "that their leg was *so heavy* they couldn't move it," OR "that one hand felt like it was *burning*," OR "that their ankle felt like it was *trapped in quicksand*," OR "that one side of their body *just went away*."

DIZZINESS AND LOSS OF BALANCE – Lots of people experience dizziness, so it is important to recognize that this is a *sudden onset of dizziness that is NOT preceded by a sudden change in head position*. This is a dizziness that just comes on without warning and is often accompanied by a loss of balance as well as the other symptoms.

It is really important for everyone to know these signs of stroke and feel confident enough to seek medical attention.

~ You may be saving someone else's life. ~

Let me give you a couple of real-life scenarios and you try to recognize the signs of the stroke:

> A.B. was at work when he developed a severe headache. He asked a colleague for an aspirin but found he was unable to open the pill bottle he was given. His right hand just would not close tightly enough over the childproof cap. So, his colleague helped him to open the pill bottle. A.B. then went to the break room to get some water to take the pills. He had to hold the water glass with his left hand, and was embarrassed when a female colleague saw him dribble some water on his shirt. He decided to go home. On the way to his car, he stumbled and dropped the car keys. A woman in the parking lot picked up his keys for him, and asked if he was okay. A.B. did not reply. It was after he crashed his car on the way home that the paramedics determined that A.B. was having a stroke.

> ———

> S.S. had finally scheduled time for lunch with friends. She had been so busy helping to plan her daughter's wedding that it was a welcomed break. S.S. was very talkative and having fun, but her friends thought it was odd that she did not eat the food on the left side of her plate. Her waiter noticed it also, and he also noticed that she was not lifting her left leg when she was walking from

the restaurant and that she seemed confused when she bumped into the door on her way out. He would have thought she was drunk, but he had not served any alcohol at their table. If you were that waiter, what would you have done?

———

I.W. was at home when her husband knew something was wrong. She had just returned from the grocery store and was unloading the groceries. She was dropping everything and kept swearing. I.W. never swore. When her husband asked if she was all right, she replied "fine, fine, f**king fine". Then, I.W. went to bed to rest. Her husband went to check on her, did the FAST test then called 911.

———

The National Stroke Association (http://www.stroke. org) uses the acronym FAST as part of their community education to help people recognize the signs of stroke. The acronym stands for **F**ace; **A**rms; **S**peech; **T**ime – providing for a quick assessment of the warning signs of stroke and emphasizing the need to call 911 immediately if a stroke is suspected.

I remember once I was giving a lecture about the need to recognize the warning signs of stroke, when someone in the audience had a stroke! Yep, right then and there a woman in the audience displayed the warning signs and the person seated next to her recognized what was happening. Oddly enough, I was the one who was hesitant to call 911. I cannot really explain why. I think I was nervous about possibly being wrong and causing a huge embarrassment. But the signs were there – and 911 was called. The paramedics arrived quickly and the woman was transported to a hospital that provided emergency treatment for her stroke. Imagine the embarrassment I would have had to face, and the guilt, if we had not called 911.

The National Institutes of Health through the National Institute of Neurological Disorders and Stroke (NINDS) also strives to educate the public about the symptoms of stroke and provides information about ongoing research and clinical trials (http://www.ninds.nih.gov/disorders/stroke.htm).

Community education about the warning signs and symptoms of stroke are the first line of attack in reducing the incidence and severity of stroke. With the multitude of resources available to learn more about the signs and symptoms of stroke, it is prudent to take the time to learn the signs. You may be the hero who seeks help for another.

~ Know Stroke. Know the Signs. Act in Time. ~

NINDS

CHAPTER FOUR

The Not So Obvious Effects of Stroke

It is rare that there is a sole survivor of a stroke. As with many illnesses and health problems, the entire family or social network of the person who had the stroke is affected. Stroke strikes across every age, ethnicity, and economic group.

> D.G. was 28 years old and had just celebrated the birth of her second child. She was busy getting the house in order before the baby woke when she had a stroke. Yes, D.G. survived the stroke but her husband, her two children and her own mother had to be survivors also. In a split second, everyone's life had changed.

> J.J. was 46 when he had his stroke. His daughter had just started college and J.J. had taken on a second job to help pay for her tuition. He had worked hard all of his adult life and did have some savings set aside, but not enough. When J.J. had his stroke, his daughter had to put aside her education, become a full-time caregiver to

her father, and hold down a full-time job. They were both survivors of the stroke.

———

S.M. was 63 and responsible for running a company that employed more than 150 people in his local community. One day, he didn't show up for work. He didn't answer phone calls and by the following day his management team was frantic. His secretary went to his home, but there was no response to her insistent banging on the door. So, she broke into the house, set off the alarm, and summoned the police. Thankfully, S.M. was still alive when the police called for an ambulance. That day, his stroke changed the lives of everyone who worked in his company.

———

The stories are endless. Each survivor has his or her own story. More than 780,000 people experience a stroke each year in the United States alone. Stroke is the leading cause of serious, long-term disability in the United States.

There are the obvious physical problems caused by a stroke: weakness and loss of sensation resulting in inability to move a body part, inability to speak or understand written or spoken words, changes in vision, etc. These are the problems that are most often addressed by rehabilitation and will receive the most attention in this book. There are also less obvious problems including, problems swallowing, loss of initiation, emotional lability, sadness and depression, loss of ego, loss of independence, problems of bowel and bladder control, relationship problems, and financial stresses.

PROBLEMS SWALLOWING – The medical term for this is Dysphagia. More than half of the survivors of brainstem stroke and one quarter of those survivors with hemiparesis have difficulty swallowing. Survivors with difficulty speaking (dysphasia or dysarthria) often have problems swallowing. To decrease the risk of aspiration (food and fluids into the lungs) it is strongly advised to have a swallowing evaluation done by a trained Speech Therapist if you notice that there is coughing or a wet-sounding voice after swallowing. With proper training and understanding of the mechanisms of swallowing, gradual improvement should be expected.

LOSS OF INITIATION – The medical term for this is Aboulia. Quite often, injuries to the brain that involve the circuitry of the Frontal Lobe and/or the Basal Ganglia can interfere with someone's ability to initiate movement, speech or even social interactions. The most common complaint from families is something like *"(S)he won't even try! I put out clothes, shoes, dinner, etc and (S)he just sits there. If I don't do everything, then nothing will get done."* Contrary to what some people may think, this lack of initiation is not intentional. The survivor of brain injury who has initiation problems may be like a car without a starter. Once the engine is started, it runs just fine... it is just difficult to start. Initiation problems combined with weakness, loss of vocalization, and depression can make rehabilitation very difficult. The key to regaining self-initiation is cognitive-rehabilitation and motivation to improve. Probably the most important intervention is to realize that this behavior is not intentional and to seek guidance on setting up a structured environment to help promote recovery. There are many resources for cognitive-rehabilitation and it may be helpful to have your physician order a neuro-psych consult.

EMOTIONAL LABILITY – The medical term for this is PseudoBulbar Affect. The stroke survivor may have an excessive display of emotion, which does not seem appropriate. They may laugh or cry for no obvious reason, or their mood may rapidly switch from laughing to crying. This can be very upsetting, even embarrassing, to the friends and family of the stroke survivor. Do not try to keep this symptom a secret from your healthcare providers, because there are treatments available. Also, learning strategies to prevent the survivor from feeling overwhelmed can be very helpful.

SADNESS AND DEPRESSION – Quite often there is a clinical depression following stroke because of a drastic change in the chemical environment of the brain. This needs to be addressed by a healthcare professional skilled in the pharmacology of the brain. There can also be severe and incapacitating sadness as one experiences loss; a loss of ego and independence, a loss of confidence, a loss of relationships, etc. This must also be addressed and the routes for recovery are many: counseling, spirituality, support groups, music, physical rehabilitation, etc. Nobody should have to go through the high, lows and plateaus alone.

LOSS OF EGO AND INDEPENDENCE - It is hard to lose one's independence. To no longer be able to use the toilet or shower independently, to prepare a meal, dress yourself, drive a car or even be able to leave the house alone is a tremendous blow to one's ego – to one's sense of self and identity. Often, the first steps to recovery include gaining independence over daily tasks. So often, I hear family members say that they "do everything" because they hate to see their father, mother, husband, wife, brother, sister *struggle*. Well, struggle is part of recovery. It is crucial to restore independence and sometimes this means people have to work really hard to put on a shirt, or they have to find a new way to be able to shower independently, etc. It is important not to let a task become defeating. I suppose that one of the hardest things about being a caregiver is learning when to let someone try it themselves and when to step in to help.

LOSS OF CONFIDENCE – It is scary to be off balance, to be out of control of your own movements. It is difficult to try and try and try again, only to not accomplish your goal. It is frightening to try and return to your place of worship, or club, or workplace. What if people do not understand you, or do not accept your disability? I remember attending a meeting once when a young man entered the group with whom I was talking. He wanted to be part of the group, but his stroke had taken away his ability to speak. I admired him tremendously when he said, "*Stroke. I hear. I try.*" With those few words, he created an acceptance for himself.

Perhaps the first step in gaining confidence is allowing others to know the reason for our limitations. As I like to say "*It is the reason, not the excuse*".

PROBLEMS WITH BOWEL AND BLADDER CONTROL - Difficulty with bowel and/or bladder control is common after stroke. It can be frustrating, embarrassing and distressing, but there are treatments available.

Poor control of the bowels or bladder can be caused by a number of changes after a stroke:

- Change of muscle tone or strength to the bowels/ bladder
- Change in sensation or feeling of need to void

- Difficulty getting to/on/off the toilet
- Difficulty dressing and undressing
- Loss of healthy bacteria in the bowels due to prolonged stress or treatment with antibiotics

The type of problems you may experience with bowel or bladder control after stroke will depend on the type of stroke you had, your age, and if you are male or female. Even though these problems can be embarrassing, it is important to have any problems evaluated and addressed. Medications, therapy, nerve stimulation, dietary changes and other treatment alternatives may be helpful.

RELATIONSHIP PROBLEMS AND FINANCIAL STRESSES – Stroke takes a toll on relationships and finances. What more can I say? In my experiences, the families that have survived and thrived after a stroke are those who keep an open line of communication and are willing to accept changes. They find new ways to share intimate time together, they establish fair expectations of one another, they communicate their feelings, and they respect one another. Learning to handle finances after a stroke is a difficult and worrisome process. Sometimes the style or standard of living may need to change, as there are new priorities for spending. Don't try to do it all alone. Ask for help. More often than not a neighbor, friend, club member, church group, or family member wants to help, but they need to be asked.

LOSS OF EMPLOYMENT – It is often possible to return to the workplace with some modifications made for accessibility or a change of job requirements. Each state also has a Division of Vocational Rehabilitation (DVR) that provides counselors to help identify a new career path or vocational opportunity.

It takes a village to raise a child and a team to recover from neurological injury. *Physiatry* — also called Physical Medicine and Rehabilitation — is a branch of medicine focused on restoring function and quality of life to people with physical or cognitive deficits due to neurological injuries, pain, physical impairments or disabilities. Physiatrists work in a multidisciplinary environment, coordinating care with physical therapists, occupational therapists, speech and language pathologists, psychologists, orthotists, and other medical and surgical specialists. As in any profession, some of these team members will be very skilled and others may not be. In my opinion, if you are not entirely satisfied with the level of care you or your loved one are receiving, then you should look for a new care provider. Especially given that most insurance-covered rehabilitation is limited and families are often left to pay out-of-pocket for many services. One must often be their own advocate to ensure that they are receiving the best standard of care. Educate yourself about the many options and services available, ask questions, and demand that your care providers be the professionals they are expected to be.

The physical recovery from stroke is only part of the story. There must also be an emotional recovery: for all of the survivors of stroke – not only the one whose brain was injured. Sometimes, it is important to go through the stages of grieving as defined by Elisabeth Kübler-Ross in 1969, and later with David Kessler. I have found that those who survive a traumatic event, such as a stroke, must go through a grieving process that is sometimes very similar to dealing with the death or loss of a loved one. This grieving process includes: Denial, Anger, Bargaining, Depression, and Acceptance.

In my opinion, it is important to grieve the loss of life, as you once knew it. The stroke took away a lot, but you survived. It is o.k. to experience the process of grieving and to acknowledge that Acceptance is part of healing. To me, acceptance doesn't mean giving up. It means being at peace with where you are at the time, while striving to be where you want to be. With the acceptance that life has changed, you will thrive. You will continue the journey through the highs, lows, and plateaus until life again is joyful and meaningful.

A lovely woman, C.M., once told me that her stroke had allowed her to have two lives: the one before her stroke and the one after. She said that she thought the one after her stroke was better because it was more loving, more accepting, and slower. She felt that in the second life she had been encouraged - not criticized; applauded for her accomplishments - not put-down for her failures. She accepted herself and she accepted her challenges. Because of that, she just kept trying to get a little bit better each year. And she did – just keep getting better, accomplishing more, and changing the lives of those around her. The stroke had not robbed her of life. It had given her a different one.

> *~ Acceptance of what has happened is the first step in overcoming the consequences of any misfortune. ~*

> *William James*

CHAPTER FIVE

HISTORY AND THE PLASTIC BRAIN

Neuroplasticity is a phenomenal feature of the nervous system that allows the nervous system to rebuild the damaged connections that have resulted in decreased abilities. Sometimes if the connections have been too severely damaged, the process of neuroplasticity allows strengthening or expansion of other connections to make up for the damaged area. This takes time and repetition.

HISTORICAL PERSPECTIVE

1890: The term "plasticity" was first introduced to the scientific literature in 1890 by a psychologist named William James. He suggested that plasticity meant "the possession of a structure weak enough to yield to an influence, but strong enough not to yield all at once." In describing the behavior of people, this would then suggest that the nervous system was capable of changing under the influence of the environment...a little bit at a time.

1913: One of the pioneers of neuroscience, Santiago Ramón y Cajal wrote:

"In adult [brain] centers the nerve paths are somewhat fixed, ended, immutable. Everything may die, nothing may be regenerated."

This writing of Cajal is mentioned in many medical neurology textbooks. **However, what most textbooks neglect to include is the other half of his statement**:

"It is for the science of the future to change, if possible, this harsh decree."

And so, the science of the future <u>has</u> changed that harsh decree. The amazing function of the human nervous system is being explored and expanded upon, with great progress being made toward understanding the plasticity and potential for change.

However, despite the suggestions of earlier researchers, up until the mid 1970's the general consensus among physicians and researchers was that brain structure and function is relatively fixed after a critical period during early childhood. It was widely believed that sensory and motor pathways that had developed during childhood could not be changed or re-routed, that brain regions served a specific and fixed function, and that no new cells could be born into the nervous system.

1990: A century after the writings of William James, President H.W. Bush and the United States Congress declared the year 1990 to mark the beginning of "Decade of the Brain". Several European countries soon followed in establishing their own funding for brain research. The congressional declaration along with The Dana Alliance for Brain Initiative stimulated funding for research into the mysteries of the nervous system.

THE BIG FINDINGS

The adult human brain has over 85 billion neurons, some receiving input from as many as about 10,000 other neurons. This number of connections is phenomenal.

Research findings gleamed from the Decade of the Brain provided the evidence that Ramón y Cajal had challenged researchers to find with his statement, *"It is for the science of the future, if possible, to change this harsh decree."* In fact, one of the most limiting dogmas of neuroscience has been the long held belief that no new nerve cells are born in the adult brain. Research advances and discoveries have demonstrated that new neurons are being created, especially in the hippocampus, a region critical for forming memories, and in the cerebral cortex. Furthermore, existing neurons are able to change their structure, connections, and chemical properties depending on the demand placed on the organism, i.e. the one using the brain.

2010: The research initiated during the Decade of the Brain (1990 – 2000) continues today with greater understanding of neuroplasticity and recovery helping to bridge the gap between research and clinical practice.

Affiliated with the Cognitive Neuroscience Section at the National Institute of Neurological Disorders and Stroke, Jordan Grafman, PhD defined four major types of neuroplasticity:

I. FUNCTIONAL MAP EXPANSION: Neurons of an active region expand or alter their activity and communication. Neuronal cells change their function, shape and connections resulting in changes in both sensory and motor signals from/to specific parts of the body. In effect, the amount of brain surface area dedicated to a specific body part changes dependent on the use and need of that body part.

II. **SENSORY REASSIGNMENT (A.K.A. CROSS-MODEL REASSIGNMENT):** When one sense is absent or diminished, cortical areas will use other sensory inputs instead. This allows one type of sensory input to entirely replace another damaged one. For example, a blind man may learn to read braille by using the sensory receptors at the fingertips to "see".

III. **COMPENSATORY MASQUERADE:** This form of plasticity allows already-constructed pathways that are adjacent to or once served a damaged area to respond to changes in the body's demands. It is this change in demand that is really critical. Basically, the brain uses alternate routes to solve a problem, IF there is opportunity given to solve the problem.

IV. **MIRROR REGION ACTIVATION (A.K.A. HOMOLOGOUS AREA ADAPTATION):** Basically, when one hemispheric region fails, the other hemisphere will take over the function. In general, the right side of the brain controls the left side of the body and vice versa. However, if regions on one side of the brain are damaged, then research indicates that regions of the other side will begin to communicate across the midline to assume the responsibilities of the injured side.

In the following Chapter Six, further discussion and examples of these four types of neuroplasticity will be provided with specific reference to recovery. Neuroplasticity, as defined by researcher Paul Bach-y-Rita, is "the adaptive capacities of the central nervous system

– its ability to modify its own structural organization and functioning.". In other words, it is the ability to learn and to change in response to the environment. *This ability to change is true of the young brain, the aging brain, and the injured brain*! It takes a lot longer in the injured brain.

Because of an increased understanding of how the brain recovers from injury, there has been a recent proliferation of new tools being introduced to the rehab market. I am so excited by these tools and really do believe that the changing landscape of rehabilitation must include tools that promote motor learning in accordance with the principles of neuroplasticity.

It is important to use the proper tool at the proper time of recovery. In Chapter Nine, the Stages of Recovery are presented. Perhaps these stages can be hastened along by the use of the appropriate rehab tools. In Chapter Eleven, I have provided an overview of electronic, robotic, bionic and mechanical tools currently available to rehabilitation, as well as emerging rehab tools.

Imagine building a house. I suppose it could be done with just a hammer... but having an array of tools in your toolbox would surely make the process easier and more successful. The same is true of recovery and building neural connections.

~ *Act as if what you do makes a difference. It does.* ~

William James

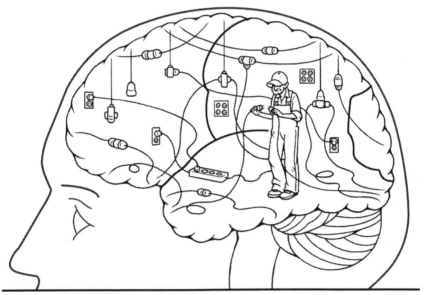

CONNECTING ELECTRICAL PATHWAYS

CHAPTER SIX

RESTORING ELECTRICAL PATHWAYS

The brain relays electrical signals. Connections between areas must be made in order for the brain to direct the concert of movement, sensation, perception, emotion, speech, vision, memory, desire, etc. The brain changes physiologically as a result of experience. The environment in which a brain operates determines to a large degree the functioning ability of that brain.

Sometimes recovery is defined by very small improvements that make a huge change in someone's life. I cannot tell you how many times I have heard statements such as, "*You know, he doesn't really need his left hand. He does fine with his right*". I think to myself... "Oh my gosh!" By denying the need for recovery, one denies the potential for recovery. Is it possible to have a full and total and complete recovery of the left hand? Maybe not. But is it possible to have a gradual continuum of improvement? I would think so. Sometimes it is small improvements. For example, being able to hold the car keys in the left hand while opening the door with the right. That is huge! But it is not on the standardized OT and PT Assessment forms, so according to many criteria, it isn't important enough. We need to change that attitude. Improvement is evidence of ongoing learning, recovery, and plasticity.

Recent advances in imaging of the brain and increasingly published evidence of the potential for reorganization of the brain following injury should change the landscape of rehabilitation. It is necessary for physicians and rehabilitation professionals to embrace a more scientific and physiological approach to neurological rehabilitation. To generalize a patient as having "hemiparesis" is a great injustice. The Stages of Recovery are presented in Chapter Nine, demonstrating that recovery is a continuum of slight changes in function, not a fixed state.

NOTES:

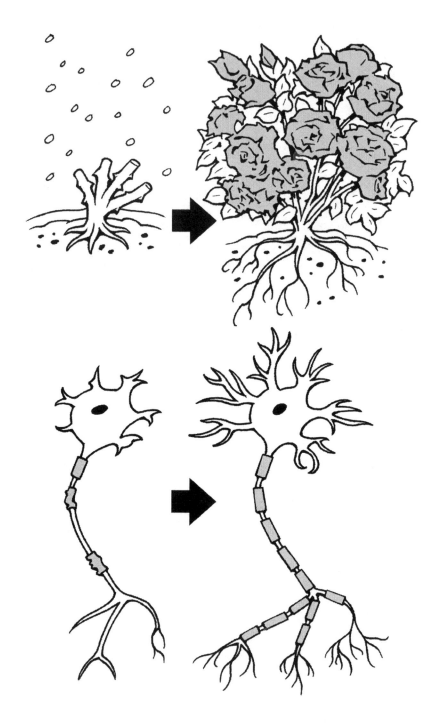

Rosebush to Neuron Analogy

In order for the various forms of cortical plasticity to occur, there must be a series of changes at the cellular level. Surviving cells must re-establish function, silent pathways become re-activated, distant regions must project toward new targets. For the purpose of discussion, I will refer to these as recovery at a cellular level. Each acts as a paving stone in establishing a viable pathway within the nervous system.

Recovery at a Cellular Level:

The analogy that I like to use is that a neuron that has been exposed to the trauma of stroke is like a rose bush in the winter. A neuron that is recovering is like a rose bush in the summer that is blooming again.

The rose bush in winter, if it has been well pruned, actually looks like it might be dead. However, it is not dead. It is conserving energy and waiting out the winter. The root bulb has pulled small rootlets inward toward the bulb, and pruning has removed the flowers and leaves, allowing the plant to survive in a harsh environment. When water, nutrients and the warm sunlight of spring return, the rose bush begins to grow again. The rootlets reach out into the soil, small limb-buds develop into branches and small flower buds give rise to beautiful flowers.

This analogy can be applied to recovering neurons.

The communicating Axon, grows out to communicate with other cells and begins to develop rootlets much like the rose does. These rootlets form terminals that provide a chemical connection to other cells. The Dendrites, which are like branches extending from the cell body, grow thicker and develop small buds that are receptors for the cell. These receptors provide a connection to other cells and allow a recovering neuron to receive chemical "instruction" from other cells in the environment. Increased blood flow to the region of recovery provides water, oxygen, and nutrients to cells in the brain. Increased action of the energy production plant (mitochondria) within each cell provides much needed energy for recovery.

NOTES:

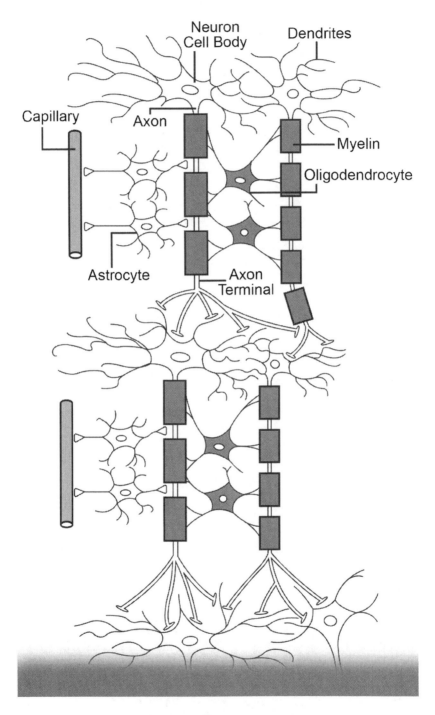

Neuron Architecture

Remember that following a stroke or brain injury, the brain environment is like a village in a war-zone. There has been a lot of damage, but not all of it is irreparable. The preceding illustration shows the key players in the central nervous system: **neurons** with their input-receiving **dendrites** and communicating **axons**, **oligodendrocytes**, **astrocytes**, and **capillaries.** When the brain is denied blood flow because of an ischemic event or when blood poisons the brain environment and creates pressure in a hemorrhagic event, all of these players can be damaged to some degree, and they can all recover to some degree.

The **neurons** are electrical cells that conduct a signal. The neurons are the business centers in the village. **Dendrites** are the branches off the neuron cell body that reach out to receive chemical input from other neurons. The **axon** is a portal that leaves the cell body to deliver chemical to the axon terminals and also, very importantly, the axon provides a conduit along which an electrical signal is conducted from the neuron cell body to the axon terminals.

> Imagine that the neurons in the upper portion of the preceding illustration are communicating with the neurons in the lower portion. The upper neurons release a chemical at the ends of the axon terminals. This chemical diffuses across a short distance to find receptors on the receiving dendrites, neuron cell body and sometimes even other axon terminals. If that chemical is excitatory, when it binds to a receptor a gate opens allowing positive ions into the cell. These positive ions excite the cell resulting in an electrical impulse that travels down the length of its axon. When the electrical signal reaches the axon terminal

it causes the release of a chemical that will bind to the receptors on the receiving dendrites and cell bodies in the next order of neurons. If that chemical is inhibitory, when it binds to a receptor a gate will open allowing negative ions into the cell. These negative ions inhibit the cell so that it cannot send the signal any further. Alternatively, if the chemical is excitatory the signal will continue to propogate. The nervous system works via an elaborate symphony of these excitatory and inhibitory signals along pathways of thousands of neurons. In a manner of speaking, damage to a portion of the pathways results in a regional electrical outage.

The **oligodendrocytes** are supporting cells that envelope the axon of the neuron and form a thick insulation called **myelin**. This myelin helps an electrical signal travel quickly along the length of an axon so that the instructions provided by the business center (neuron) reach their destination without delay.

The **astrocytes** are also supporting cells that are the delivery trucks that deliver supplies to the business center. These cells latch one end-foot onto a capillary and the other onto the neuron to allow oxygen and nutrition to diffuse from the blood to the neuron. This is really important, because blood is actually toxic to neurons when it comes in direct contact with the neuron cell wall. Astrocytes also work as the cleanup crew, keeping the environment for the neuron free of toxins.

The **capillaries** are the small blood vessels that act as the roads into the village to allow supplies to be brought in and delivered. The brain environment has a high demand for oxygen and nutrition so these supply routes are critical.

Rebuilding after the war is not just a matter of getting the business center up and running again. Electrical lines need to be restored and insulated, supplies need to be delivered, roads need to be reopened and a customer/destination needs to be re-established. The same is true in rebuilding the nervous system. This process can take time and requires persistence, since there are bound to be some highs, lows, and plateaus during the recovery.

RECOVERY AT A CELLULAR LEVEL

- Axonal sprouting
- Distributed myelination
- Dendritic sprouting
- Increased receptor density
- Altered neurochemical stores
- Increased vascular collaterals

AXONAL SPROUTING – the axon grows additional terminals so that it can communicate with a greater number of other neurons. When a neuron is excited, it sends an electrical signal down the axon that causes the release of a chemical at the axon terminal. This chemical then binds to receptors on the receiving cell and either excites, or inhibits that cell (depending on the type of chemical released).

DISTRIBUTED MYELINATION – the oligodendrocytes form denser and more complete myelin to optimize the insulation of the axon, helping signals to be conducted more quickly.

DENDRITIC SPROUTING – more dendritic branches form, allowing there to be more area for incoming axon terminals to make a connection.

INCREASED RECEPTOR DENSITY – the dendrites and cell bodies of neurons distribute more receptors into the membrane walls so that the cell is really ready for the chemical that is going to be released by the axons.

ALTERED NEUROCHEMICAL STORES – neurons begin to increase their storage of neurochemicals to support an increased number of axon terminals. In some cases, the neuron can actually modify the type of chemical being made.

INCREASED VASCULAR COLLATERALS – areas of the brain that are recovering and being used develop elaborate capillary beds so that there is plenty of blood supply making oxygen and nutrition available.

These processes can take time. The brain has the remarkable ability to direct populations of neurons to resume responsibility for a function they had prior to the injury OR assume a new responsibility. When recovery utilizes neuron populations adjacent to the region of injury less time is required than when recovery utilizes neuron populations that may be distant to the injury or even on the other side of the brain. Changes in neural activity, equate to changes in sensory and motor function. This ability to change is neuroplasticity.

I briefly touched on the four types of cortical neuroplasticity in the previous chapter. Following are just a few examples from the research literature:

I. **FUNCTIONAL MAP EXPANSION:** neurons of an active region expand or alter their activity and communication.

The nervous system has a somatotopic organization. What this means is that certain cell populations are organized to represent certain body parts. For example, as I strike the keys of the keyboard to type, my brain knows the precise location of each of my fingers because each finger has an established group of cells that perceive sensation. Another group of related cells command the motor activity of striking the keyboard. The sensory and motor contributions are well coordinated because my brain calls into action only the cells needed for the task. Other sets of cells, perhaps those designated for my forehead and mouth, remain quiet since I don't really need them for typing.

Following a stroke, some of the brain cells that control the hand may die; some may be injured or have gone silent. If the hand is not used after the stroke, surviving cells no longer have a job. Reorganization can occur, such that the adjacent regions dedicated to the forehead and mouth begin to expand their boundaries and encompass some of the cells that used to be dedicated to the hand. Therapists and stroke survivors witness this when the survivor opens their mouth and contorts their face when trying to exercise the paretic hand. The exciting thing about recovery is that cortical reorganization is plastic and changeable. Reorganization is dependent on activity and use.

> Cortical reorganization was measured in stroke survivors who were between three and nine months post-stroke and participating in a trial of Constraint-Induced Movement Therapy (CIMT). The therapy required that each survivor participate in 10 consecutive weekdays of intensive upper extremity therapy and that they wear a mitt over their unaffected hand for at least 90% of all waking hours during the two-week period. Using Transcranial Magnetic Stimulation (TMS) as a tool to measure brain activity, researchers were able to demonstrate

41

an enlargement in the active area on the same side of the brain as the injury in the region dedicated to a finger extensor muscle (FDC). This increased active area of the brain correlated with improvements in grip force. The increased brain activity and improved grip force were maintained at a 4-month follow-up evaluation. (Sawaki et al. 2008)

II. SENSORY REASSIGNMENT: when one sense is absent or diminished, cortical areas will use other sensory inputs.

It has long been held that the brain has distinct regions dedicated to the senses: the occipital lobe processes vision, the olfactory lobe processes smell, the parietal lobe processes touch, the temporal lobe processes hearing, while the sense of taste is processed by the brainstem and temporal lobe. Until recently, it was believed that these functions were fixed to these specific brain regions. Yet, intuitively many of us recognize that a blind-man reading Braille is actually using the sense of touch to substitute for vision. Years ago, I had a client who had NO sensory awareness of his leg. Like many stroke survivors he walked slowly and looked down to see his foot. That is, until he relearned walking by "listening" to the sound of his heel-strike. Perhaps, he had substituted sound for proprioception.

> Paul Bach-y-Rita devoted much of his research career to the study of Sensory Substitution. A human-machine interface having an array of electrical stimulators on the tongue has been demonstrated to provide 'visual acuity' for the blind. A small camera mounted on the forehead scans the environment and then sends an array of electrical stimulation to the tongue, allowing the person to perceive their surroundings using the stimulation pattern they feel on the tongue

(Sampio, Maris, Bach-y-Rita 2001). Likewise, patients who have lost their sense of balance due to injury to the vestibular system (inner ear organ that detects self-motion) have been able to regain their balance using an array of electrical stimulation to the tongue. When they begin to fall right, the right side of the tongue tingles, letting them know to correct their balance. Likewise, a fall to the left, forward and backward is detected. They learn to substitute sensation on the tongue for vestibular function (Bach-y-Rita and Kercel 2003; Danilov, et al. 2007)

III. COMPENSATORY MASQUERADE: more than one way for the brain to approach the problem.

There are diffuse and redundant pathways throughout the central nervous system. Often pathways that were used during initial learning, become silent or infrequently used after a task is well learned. Imagine a highway that has a frontage road running adjacent to it. Most traffic takes the highway. But, if for some reason the highway becomes blocked, then the frontage road will provide a very good alternative route.

> Several interconnected areas of the cortex project to the brainstem and the spinal cord to control the muscles of the legs and arms. This redundancy often allows for significant recovery. In contrast, there is only one route from the cortex for fine control of the hand and fingers. With regard to control of the arm and hand, primate studies have demonstrated that damaging the axons from the cortex to the spinal cord results in paralysis of the hand and synergies in movement of the wrist, elbow and shoulder. However, with demand for use and practice the primates can relearn reaching and grasp using pathways that originate in the

brainstem (Lawrence and Kuypers 1968). If not all of the descending axons are damaged, it is also possible for adjacent regions of the brain to take over the controls. For example, when learning new motor tasks, the brain uses multiple areas such as the supplementary motor cortex, the premotor cortex and the primary motor cortex. However, once a movement is proficient and skilled it is often controlled by only a small set of neurons in the primary motor cortex. If cells from the region are injured, then cells from the supplementary motor area may become reactivated and help "relearn" the movement (Roland et al. 1980).

IV. MIRROR REGION TAKE-OVER: when one hemisphere of the brain fails the other will take over.

The human brain has two halves. Typically, the right half controls the left side of the body. Likewise the left half of the brain controls the right side of the body. Also, the left half of the brain controls our ability to speak, while the right side has more control over perception of our environment. Historically, it was believed that this half-brain specialization was hard-wired and not really able to change. We now know that this is not the case. It is possible for the undamaged side of the brain to "learn" the function of the damaged side. - this can take a long time and require a lot of hard work.

> Children who have suffered extensive injury to one side of the brain often show remarkable recovery of both sensation and movement on the side of the body that the injured brain would have controlled. Functional MRI studies have demonstrated that the undamaged side of the brain, takes over the function of the damaged side. (Holloway et al. 2000)

While it has been generally believed that this ability of the undamaged side of the brain reflects the high capacity of the immature brain for cerebral reorganization, studies have also demonstrated this phenomenon in the brain of adult stroke survivors. Imaging of the functional anatomy of the brain during movement shows brain activity on both sides of the brain during recovery of hand movement with a predominance of activity on the undamaged side of the brain (Chollet et al. 1991).

Using a special type of brain imaging (functional MRI) researchers studied seven stroke survivors who had lost their ability to speak following the stroke and then regained their speech. They found that in the stroke survivors who regained speech, there was increased activity in new speech areas on the right side of the brain. Hence, the right half of the brain had taken over the function for the damaged left side. Survivors with the best language recovery actually showed activation of speech centers on both sides of the brain. (Cao Y, et al. 1999)

The challenge for rehabilitation is to understand how to optimize the use of neuronal circuits that may be damaged or silent, but not dead. By applying research and the concepts of motor learning to rehabilitation, the stroke survivor should be given the opportunity and encouragement for an ongoing continuum of recovery.

~ *Your brain - every brain - is a work in progress.*
It is 'plastic.' From the day we're born to the day we
die, it continuously revises and remodels, improving or
slowly declining, as a function of how we use it. ~

Michael Merzenich

45

NOTES:

CHAPTER SEVEN

"PLATEAU" IS NOT A 4-LETTERED WORD

How many of you or your loved ones have been told that "your recovery has **plateaued**"? Has that been used as a Good word, or a Bad word? Often it sounds like a bad word – like something terrible has happened. Often it means the end of insurance-covered rehabilitation. Nobody wants to hear that they have *"plateaued"*!

Let's think of a different meaning for the word. If you are climbing a mountain – perhaps Mount Everest- don't you think it would be nice to reach a plateau? It would be a nice level place where you can pitch a tent, get a bit of rest and prepare for the next big ascent.

In this case, a plateau is not a bad thing. A plateau is a point in the recovery when the nervous system has reached a stable state. The nervous system is consolidating its' learning and preparing for the next stage of recovery. In recovery, there will be highs, lows, and plateaus. In many ways it is like climbing a mountain. In order to move past the plateau, one must continue to accept and face new challenges.

In rehabilitation terms, a plateau is when measurable change is difficult to document. Often, it is when insurance stops paying for rehabilitation appointments or when the therapist cannot think of new exercises. Sometimes a new tool is required or a new set of exercises needed to move past a plateau. Sometimes, the survivor reaches a point in recovery where they are content and do not really see a need to move past that point. That is o.k. also, as long the individual has made that decision, but remember that damage to brain can affect executive functions such that decision making and initiation becomes difficult for the survivor. This is when they need a family member or friend to believe in them and advocate for them.

There are no rules as to how long someone may be at a plateau in their recovery. Sometimes one spends only a brief time at a plateau, sometimes they are there for years. Each stroke is different and each recovery is per the individual. I want to stress that ongoing improvement is possible, but it requires time, finances, a supportive environment and a personal drive to improve.

The research findings of Dr. Paul Bach-y-Rita (Chapter Six) have intrigued me for many years. His pursuit to understand and explain plasticity – especially sensory substitution – had a personal component. Norman Doidge tells the story of how in 1959 Paul Bach-y-Rita's father, Pedro, had a very severe stroke and then a dramatic recovery. After a rather ordinary short burst of rehabilitation, the family was told that Pedro had no hope of recovery, i.e. he had plateaued. Pedro went home with his other son, George, who knew nothing about post-stroke recovery. Using an exercise regime that turned normal day-to-day life experiences into exercise, Pedro (with his son's help) began the long path toward recovery. They struggled along through each day, through each repetition and gradually improvement dawned. Despite an extensive brain injury from his stroke, Pedro Bach-y-Rita had a near full recovery. He returned to teaching, married again and resumed travelling and hiking. All of this long before researchers had begun to talk openly about neuroplasticity and the importance of a sensory rich environment.

> T.N. lived with his wife following his stroke. Their day was very routine. He would wake and she would help him dress. Once dressed, he would use his wheelchair to go to the dining table for breakfast. Following breakfast, his wife would clean the dishes while T.N. read his newspapers. While his wife took care of all of the household needs, T.N. would wait in his wheelchair...and so the day continued. T.N. would complain about being cold and worry that his muscles were getting stiff, but the most exercise he ever had was transferring from the wheelchair to toilet! We made a few simple changes that enriched his sensory environment. He began standing at the table (wheelchair behind and wall to his side) while his wife did the dishes. With his wife standing nearby for safety, he stood while brushing his teeth and shaving. He became responsible for writing the checks while they managed the household bills together. Then, he enrolled in an Adapted Physical Education class at the local community college and began socializing with new friends and began walking short distances and exercising again. There were highs, lows and plateaus, but T.N. continued to improve and gain more independence as he lived a more rich and fulfilling life. His goals now are to be able to regain his driving license and to take his wife on a vacation.

It is true that the fastest improvements are generally seen within the first six months following a stroke. That may be due to decreasing inflammation in the brain environment and also the fact that most therapy is provided during those first few months. Continuing improvement and recovery is possible long after the first six months or even a year. I have heard from people eleven years, sixteen years, even twenty-two years post-stroke who have gained new abilities or met a goal they had set for themselves. Often, what they needed was the right tool and a therapist or team who believed in them. In Chapter Eleven, I will introduce some of the tools that I have found to be useful in promoting recovery.

> F.G. began learning to walk while wearing the rigid plastic ankle brace (AFO) that he had been fit with while still in the hospital. He walked with a stiff left leg that he swung sideways at the hip to advance forward (circumduction). We began to retrain his walking pattern by changing his AFO so that it had a flexible ankle joint and a flexible footplate. He began learning to bend his knee during walking. A few months later, he was able to use the Tibion Bionic Leg. His left leg strength improved tremendously! We were then able to introduce a Walk-Aide system to help him clear his left foot while walking. He now had the hip flexion, the knee bend, and the foot clearance critical to a healthy walking pattern. After about 1 year, he stopped using the Walk-Aide and only wore a lightweight volleyball ankle brace when walking. Last time I saw him, his goal was to run again!

One further point that I would like to stress, is that plateaus sometimes happen because medical practice or associated technology isn't available to facilitate further recovery.

> D.Y. learned to walk following her stroke, but the walking pattern was not good. In compensation for the weakened leg, she learned to hike the hip and land on her toes, forcing the knee into

hyperextension with each step. Her walking was too slow to be useful and because of back pain she resorted to using a Segway to get around. Years after her initial stroke, D.Y. began to use the KickStart by Cadence Biomedical. Now, with the orthosis, she walks everywhere and has even started taking ballroom dance classes with her husband.

As the saying goes "necessity is often the mother of invention." Many times in my career it has been the stroke survivor or the loved one whom has designed a tool or treatment approach that helps to move past the plateau.

C.B. had severe vision problems following her stroke. Two ophthalmologists said that her optical nerve was irreversibly damaged resulting in a disabling and distorted vision that she would just have to learn to live with. Furthermore, one of these professionals was quite condescending and said not to spend too much time on vision therapy – because it wouldn't help. C.B.'s husband wasn't willing to accept that and developed a program on his laptop that allowed C.B. to practice following a small red cursor across the screen. It took a lot of time and a lot of practice, but her field of view has increased and the two eyes now see the same thing in the same place.

Even the most accomplished skill requires ongoing practice. The famous cellist, Pablo Casals, who practiced playing almost daily until his death at age 96, was once asked *why* he continued to practice.

Casals replied, *"Because I think I am making some progress."*

~ *Success is often achieved by a series of very small steps.* ~

```
┌─────────────────────────────┐
│      Injury to the          │
│      Nervous System         │
└─────────────────────────────┘
              │
              ▼
┌─────────────────────────────┐
│    Abnormal or Absent        │
│        Movement              │
│                              │
│ Paresis / Altered Muscle     │
│ Tone / Non-Use               │
└─────────────────────────────┘
              │
              ▼
┌─────────────────────────────┐
│       Movement               │
│    Attempted Less            │
│                              │
│ Cortical Reorganization /    │
│ Muscle Atrophy /             │
│ Synaptic Ineffectiveness     │
└─────────────────────────────┘
              │
              ▼
┌─────────────────────────────┐
│   Secondary Problems         │
│        Develop               │
│                              │
│ Generalized weakness /       │
│ Deconditioning /             │
│ Contractures / Neglect       │
└─────────────────────────────┘
```

CHAPTER EIGHT

Injury To The Brain and Then What

When the brain is injured, there is the initial injury and then a cascade of problems following that injury. The initial effect of a stroke is disrupted flow of blood to the brain: either due to a clot, or due to rupture of a blood vessel. Regardless of the specific mechanism, some brain cells begin to die. As these neuronal cells die, they release the chemical content of their cell body. These chemicals are toxic to surrounding cells and also create an environment of waste products and inflammation.

INJURY TO THE NERVOUS SYSTEM

It is important to appreciate that not all of the cells in the region of the stroke die. A large number of cells survive, but go into a state of "shut-down"; a low energy state to ensure survival. Other cells that are not directly in the region of the stroke have lost communication with/from the dead or damaged cells. They in turn go silent.

ABNORMAL OR ABSENT MOVEMENT

So now, the individual has survived the initial insult but is left with the deficits caused by a nervous system that is no longer conducting signals or communicating correctly. Movement becomes very difficult. There may be no movement on the affected side of the body, no sensation, no speech, no control of volition, OR movement, sensation, speech, etc. may be altered.

PARESIS

Generally, the terms "paresis" or "hemiparesis" are used to describe the weakness following a stroke. Paresis means weakness of voluntary movement and/or partial loss of voluntary control of the limbs, vocal cords, eye muscles, etc. Hemiparesis refers to a weakness on one side of the body.

ALTERED MUSCLE TONE

In addition to weakness, the stroke survivor may also experience altered muscle tone. SPASTICITY is a velocity-dependent stretch reflex that causes muscles to reflexively tighten in response to a quick stretch. Spasticity can really interfere with recovery of movement, because every time one muscle group is shortened, its opposing muscle group is stretched. Sometimes, quick stretch of one muscle group results in reflex shortening and CLONUS develops. The best example of clonus is the shaking or "ankle beat" of the foot. Remember, the muscles of the ankle work in opposition to one another. If the gastrocnemius (on the back of the calf) is stretched, a sensory signal is sent to the spinal cord exciting the spinal motor neurons that send a signal to shorten the muscle. But, if the gastrocnemius shortens, then there will be a stretch to the tibialis muscle (on the front of the calf). The sensory signal from the tibialis will travel to the spinal cord exciting the spinal motor neurons that send a signal to shorten that muscle. But... when the tibialis shortens, the gastrocnemius is stretched... and the ankle just keeps beating along. Normally, this stretch reflex will have been inhibited or regulated by a descending signal from the higher brain, but due to the injury the descending signal is not making it down to the spinal cord neurons. One simple trick to interrupt this clonus is to touch the heel of the foot. The sensory signal from the heel will interrupt that reflex loop at the spinal cord and stop the clonus.

Another form of abnormal muscle tone is HYPERTONICITY. In this case, the muscles get stiff making it difficult to move a joint. This abnormal tone is a result of the motor neurons in the spinal cord getting a little too excited and not being quieted or regulated by a descending signal from the higher brain. Sometimes, hypertonicity results from motor centers in the brainstem sending an excitatory signal down to the spinal cord. For example, when one moves from sitting to standing, there is an excitation of the vestibular system, which is the balance mechanism of the inner ear. This system sends an excitatory signal to the spinal cord causing the legs to straighten and the arm to bend. Normally, this signal is well balanced by a convergence of other signals related to what one plans to do, what one has done before, and the current environment conditions and goal. After a stroke, descending signals from the higher brain don't have good convergence and lower brain centers have too strong of an influence. This generally results in the hemi-paretic pattern of walking with a stiff leg and bent elbow.

Non-Use

The paresis and altered muscle tone can result in a non-use of the limb. If there is also an abnormal sensory awareness, the survivor may actually neglect the body part. Sometimes, the survivor cannot feel their arm or leg on the side of paresis. In severe cases, they do not even recognize that the body part belongs to them. It is very difficult to learn to move a body part that you cannot feel. For that reason, much of therapy should focus on both the sensory and motor rehabilitation.

MOVEMENT ATTEMPTED LESS

Following the stroke, because movement is so difficult and sensation is often abnormal, movement is attempted less often. When movement is attempted less, the brain begins to reorganize itself around the area of injury and decreased communication. Synapses become less effective and muscles begin to atrophy. Now, the survivor has not only the effects of the stroke injury to overcome, but they also have a cascade of problems related to the non-use that must also be overcome.

CORTICAL REORGANIZATION

The brain will begin to re-designate surviving cells for other functions. For example, if the arm is no longer being used, the surviving cells in the brain that used to communicate signals for motor control and sensation of the arm may start being used for control of the facial muscles instead. Often, when a stroke survivor is beginning to learn to open their paretic hand, they will exert great effort and also open their mouth! This is an example of cortical reorganization...a melding together of the regions of the brain that represent the hand and the face. It is important not to discourage the movements of the mouth. Ignore them and continue to encourage the hand. Cortical reorganization is a plastic property of the brain. It is continually changing based on use.

SYNAPTIC INEFFECTIVENESS

Disuse or non-use can also result in synaptic ineffectiveness. A synapse is the junction at which one brain cell (neuron) communicates with another neuron. We also have synapses at the muscle where a neuron from the spinal cord sends a message to the muscle fibers. When a neural pathway is not used frequently, or when a muscle is not exercised, these synapses become less effective. Imagine that a neuron from the spinal cord is trying to send a signal to contract and move a muscle. A healthy neuron may have a synaptic terminal kind of like a sprinkler head. When the signal gets to the end of the nerve, it is spread out over multiple terminals with a disperse excitation of the muscle. So, like a sprinkler head, a single source can actually provide nourishment and energy to a wide area. Now, imagine that the sprinkler head gets clogged with sludge and the water is only leaving a couple of the openings in the sprinkler head. Not all of the grass is getting water and it begins to wither. The same is true of our muscles and ineffective synapses. Even though the brain may be trying to send a signal to move the muscles, the signal is weak and not enough muscle fibers get the signal. Also, the muscles may be atrophied and lacking bulk. The net result is an injured nervous system and a weakened muscular system. However, the more a signal is sent down the same pathway, the more robust the signal, the more effective the synapse and the stronger the muscle.

MUSCLE ATROPHY

Muscle fibers also have a very dynamic ability to change and adjust their physical and functional properties in response to the demand placed on the muscle. Inactivity combined with neurological injury results in an increase in intramuscular fat with a rapid loss of muscle mass and strength. This weakness combined with an overactive stretch reflex and excessive co-contraction increasingly complicate efforts to move.

SECONDARY PROBLEMS DEVELOP

Often recovery is impeded by not only the brain injury but also the secondary problems that develop due to decreased activity and movement.

GENERALIZED WEAKNESS AND DECONDITIONING

Weight gain and poor cardiovascular endurance further contribute to the problems one must face during recovery. Establishing an exercise routine and changing dietary habits is often a critical part of recovery. Moving the body post-stroke is very difficult, moving an over-weight body is even more difficult. Another thing to take into consideration is that many stroke survivors develop sleep apnea (difficulties breathing during sleep), in part because the muscles of the airway become weak. Your doctor can request a sleep study if it seems relevant.

CONTRACTURES

A muscle that has hypertonicity or one that has not been used for a period of time is vulnerable to contractures, which involve physical shortening of the muscle. The muscle actually looses some of its muscle fibers, becoming shorter and weaker. It is possible to reverse this shortening with active exercise and stretching but it takes a long time. It is therefore, really important to maintain good range of motion at all joints and have good muscle length and flexibility to optimize the potential for ongoing recovery.

NEGLECT

Injury to the nervous system that results in non-use and abnormal sensory awareness of a limb can lead to neglect of the limb. In severe cases, the survivor may sit on their hand or get it caught in the wheelchair wheel and not even notice. They may only shave one half of their face, completely unaware that they even have another side still to shave. They may only put their coat on one arm, not realizing that they have another arm to still get in the coat. Neglect does improve over time, but it is generally easier if early rehab focuses on establishing a good awareness of the body. Extra attention should be directed toward the paretic side of the body.

The fundamental concept is to *reverse* the flow diagram shown at the beginning of this chapter. To reverse muscle weakness, demand more of the muscles. Any movement that can be made should be rewarded and practiced. As one movement becomes easier then attempt a new movement. Stretching and massage should be incorporated into the exercise routine. Aerobic and resistive exercise training strategies are also beneficial for patients with chronic stroke.

A higher demand of the muscles will require greater synaptic effectiveness and will also provide sensory drive to the nervous system. Improved synaptic effectiveness and evolving sensory awareness will reduce abnormal muscle tone and allow muscles to move more easily. A limb that is repeatedly moved will help establish a stronger cortical representation and promote cellular recovery and neural plasticity. Exercise needs to be a lifelong commitment, not just a short-term rehabilitation phase. Recovery does not take place in a matter of weeks; it can take years.

In my opinion, the conventional rehabilitation phase of stroke recovery is too short. We cannot accomplish enough in a short period of time unless there is a high degree of repetition and repeatability. The number of visits and the length of visits often limit therapists. Energy, finances, and the need for help from another person often limit survivors. To benefit from the highest repetition and consistency of practice, one may need to find the tools that best fit the task requirement at each phase of recovery. We will address this more in the subsequent chapters. Also, ongoing recovery will require ongoing effort to recover. Often survivors will need help finding resources outside of the insurance-based rehabilitation, since initiation, self-confidence, speech, etc are often affected by the stroke. As the survivor recovers, they will need less help. Resource options would include Adapted Physical Education Classes available at many community colleges, gym memberships, group exercise programs, private-pay with personal trainers or therapists, participation in research trials and personal goal setting and challenges.

> R.G. survived a ruptured blood vessel in his brain. He learned to walk again with a cane but it was painfully slow. So, he challenged himself to improve. Each day he went to the park and walked a small paved loop around the park. It was about ¼ mile distance and the first time it took him over one hour to complete one loop. But, he walked the same path everyday and set a goal to decrease his time by a few seconds each day.

The last time I saw him, he reported that he was able to complete the loop in about 10 minutes, so he was now walking 4 loops each day!

Many times, I hear from family members that they do not want to see their wife/husband/child struggle and so they do too much to help. It is important to remember that learning requires practice and mistakes. Sometimes, one needs to be patient and provide a safe environment for the stroke survivor to practice and learn. It is important not to treat the survivor like a child. Talk to one another. Establish a routine. Set reasonable expectations and encourage recovery.

S.H. was a kindergarten teacher and her stroke took away her ability to speak. It pained her husband to see her struggling for words and he wanted to help, so he began to do all of the speaking for her. About two months after her stroke, I was working with S.H. and asked her husband a series of questions about her rehabilitation. Suddenly, she shouted "No, No, No" and wagged her finger toward me. Then she clapped her chest and said "Me". So, I redirected my questions – slowly, clearly, succinctly toward her. She was able to nod, smile and occasionally say "yes" or "no" in response. When she needed help, she looked to her husband, nodded and said "Now". He then filled in the gaps of information. I learned a lot from S.H. She began to bring in children's books with lots of pictures and she could tell me a few words about each picture. She didn't speak well, but she did communicate. When I moved to Holland, I had to try and speak Dutch in our small community. In some ways, I felt like S.H., trying to grasp the correct word and trying to communicate. I saw S.H. about 5 years after we had worked together and she spoke beautifully. Although she had not yet returned to teaching, she was a teacher's assistant and she volunteered at the local library having children read to her. I have no doubt, that at the writing of this book, she has only continued to regain her power of speech.

We must make mistakes in order to learn. We must move in order to experience movement. It is not in being told what to do that we become masters of our skill, but in doing. When someone is learning to move again, they do not always need instruction. Sometimes all that is needed is someone else to help keep them safe and to help encourage them as they try to experience movement. Remember, start with what you can do ~ then do more of that until you can do something more.

~ *Tell me and I forget. Teach me and I may remember. Involve me and I learn.* ~

Benjamin Franklin

CHAPTER NINE

STAGES IN THE CONTINUUM OF RECOVERY

Often, the most rapid improvement period following a stroke is during the first few months. This is generally associated with decreasing inflammation as the body cleans up waste products and debris from the damaged region of the brain. As the environment is recovering, surviving neurons begin to communicate again. This phase of recovery is generally not considered to be due solely to neuroplasticity, but rather to a general awakening of the nervous system.

Too often, stroke survivors and their families are led to believe that ALL of the recovery has taken place during the first few months following the stroke. This is an entirely incorrect belief! Yes, the most rapid rate of improvement is during this time, but the nervous system and muscular system – when properly challenged and trained – will be capable of so much more.

STAGES OF RECOVERY

The process of recovery from stroke usually follows a series of stages. In 1951 a psychologist, Thomas E. Twitchell, published a highly detailed report describing the pattern of motor recovery following a stroke. His observations were based on the recovery pattern of 121 patients: 118 of whom had a stroke due to a blood clot interrupting blood flow in one of the major cerebral vessels, and 3 of whom had a bleed. All of the patients presented with weakness and sensory loss on one side of the body. His observations included the following:

- *At onset of hemiplegia, the arm is more involved than the leg, and eventual motor recovery in the leg occurs earlier, and is more complete, than in the arm*
- *Most recovery takes place in the first three months and only minor additional recovery occurs after six months post onset*

These observations have, in part, shaped the focus of rehab over the past 60 years. It is not at all uncommon to hear a doctor or other health care provider tell families that most recovery takes place in the first six months. That is true, but remember that most of the swelling and irritation of the brain decreases allowing the brain to recover some function. Also, in the first few months, patients tend to have the most intensive rehabilitation.

Twitchell's observations and predictions were accurate but somewhat limited by the emergency care of stroke and the rehabilitation tools available at the time. Unfortunately, they also resulted in a self-fulfilling prophecy: *"Since improvement is not expected, let's not work toward more improvement."*

To this I say, BUNK!! Our knowledge base has increased, the tools available for rehabilitation have proliferated, and our society has come to expect more.

During the 1960's, a Swedish Physical Therapist, Signe Brunnstrom also described the process of recovery following stroke-induced hemiplegia and developed her own approach to therapy. The Brunnstrom Approach, emphasizes the importance of encouraging movement within the synergistic pattern of movement that evolves post-stroke. *As the stroke survivor improves, the exercises change*. This approach encourages development of flexor and extensor synergies (patterns of movement) during early recovery. As the nervous system recovers, then progressive exercises will promote a progression into smooth voluntary control of movements. Brunnstrom believed that no reasonable training method should be left untried.

Often the leg and the arm are at different stages of recovery. Sometimes a survivor may quickly progress from one stage to another and sometimes there may be years between the progressions. What inspires hope is the potential for ongoing recovery.

BRUNNSTROM'S STAGES OF MOTOR RECOVERY

Modified from Brunnstrom's Stages of Motor Recovery (1966)

STAGE ONE: No voluntary movement of the limb can be initiated.

No spasticity noted.

STAGE TWO: Basic limb synergies begin to appear.

Spasticity is mild.

STAGE THREE: Basic limb synergies seen with any effort to move.

Spasticity is increased.

STAGE FOUR: Some movements begin to deviate from basic synergies.

Spasticity begins to decrease.

STAGE FIVE: Relative independence from the basic limb synergies.

Spasticity is mild.

STAGE SIX: Individual isolated joint movements become possible.

Spasticity is negligible.

~

In the following discussion, a FEW examples of how the body may be responding at each stage of recovery will be provided. I will focus on the evolution of the flexor synergy of the arm and the extensor synergy of the leg. These are by no means the only movements or movement combinations possible, but they are the more common. Every stroke is different. However, there are basic commonalities seen in the movement challenges resulting from the stroke. What I hope you can appreciate is that there is a continuum of recovery with each phase setting the stage for the next.

~

STAGE ONE:

This is immediately following the storm. The brain is in a state of shock. There is swelling, and cellular debris, and a toxic environment.

The patient has survived the stroke and now presents with a varying degrees of symptoms ranging from a mild to total loss of "voluntary movement" on the affected side. The muscles are flaccid, heavy, and seemingly lifeless. Sensation is often lost or severely diminished. Sometimes, the survivor is unable to feel or even find his or her own arm, hand, leg or foot. If the speech centers of the brain have been affected then the survivor will have lost the freedom of written and spoken communication.

Stage One is about surviving the storm. Generally, therapy is directed at passive range of motion and learning to move well enough to be taken care of by others.

STAGE TWO:

Basic limb synergies begin to appear. Spasticity develops but is mild. In this stage, the nervous system is beginning to become active again. In general, lower brain areas assume dominance for the stereotypic patterns/synergies of movement. Voluntary movements require use of the cortex – higher brain – therefore control of voluntary movements is minimal, since this is most often the region of the nervous system injured by a stroke.

UPPER EXTREMITY: ARM AND HAND

In Stage One and Two, the shoulder is generally *subluxed*. This means that it has slipped from the joint. Passive Range of Motion can be painful if the person performing the range of motion does not also move the scapula (shoulder blade) with the arm. *It is very important to avoid pain!* Range of motion is important but must include rotation of the scapula if the arm is brought to more than a 60 degree angle to the body. In general, there is no voluntary control of the shoulder at this stage of recovery.

The elbow may assume a slight flexion with a bit of resistance to being passively straightened. In general, there is no voluntary control of the elbow at this stage of recovery. Passive range of motion to maintain FULL elbow motion is very important at this stage, but the elbow should always be supported when being straightened so that the shoulder is not pulled away from the socket and injured.

The hand may assume slight flexion of the fingers and a reflexive grip may cause this flexion to tighten when the hand is held or instructed to move. In general, there is no voluntary control of the hand at this stage of recovery. Often, the stroke survivor reports NO awareness of touch to the hand or severely impaired sensation. It is recommended to have someone massage and stretch the stroke survivor's hand several times daily. This helps to maintain the range of motion of the joints and also provide some sensory stimulation to the hand during this stage of recovery.

LOWER EXTREMITY: LEG, ANKLE AND FOOT

Much like the shoulder, the hip joint is generally very lax during this stage of recovery and may even be subluxed. There is a loss of stabilization at the hip and in general no voluntary movement of the leg. The stroke survivor requires assistance to move at every joint of the leg.

During this stage of recovery, there may be very slight voluntary control over the hip and knee when the stroke survivor is lying down on his or her back, but there is no control of the ankle or foot. The foot may begin to assume a "toes-down" position. It is really important NOT to allow the Achilles tendon on the back of the ankle to shorten. For this reason, resting splints, night splints, and ankle braces are often provided.

The leg cannot really support any body weight. There is not enough muscular control. Often the survivor is fit with a rigid ankle brace to stabilize the foot and ankle so that they have at least some control during standing. When the survivor is assisted into a standing position they generally rely on the ankle brace and the inherent stability of the joints. The knee may assume a slightly locked position and the pelvis retracts or rotates backward. Often, there is a slight excitatory signal from the brainstem that causes the leg muscles to stiffen the leg into extension and provide support against the force of gravity.

Standing is important, however it is very important to remember that the brace provided during Stage Two of recovery is NOT the brace that is going to help the survivor learn to walk in the subsequent phases of recovery. The initial fabrication of a brace for standing should include the potential to add a joint for ankle motion once the survivor is ready to begin gait training.

STAGE THREE:

Basic limb synergies are seen with any effort to move the limb. Increase in spasticity. This is often a very frustrating stage of recovery as the stroke survivor begins to be able to voluntarily make slight movements but the movements are not yet functional or helpful. Furthermore, efforts to move often result in increased spasticity and resistance to movement. In general, movements are predominantly driven by the motor control of the brainstem and not of the higher brain. Those brainstem pathways and spinal reflexes remain unchecked by the higher brain, causing tone to increase. Nonetheless this is the beginning of recovery of movement. This is the stage of recovery during which one must identify what they _can do_ and then perform high repetitions of that movement, gradually refining the movement over time as they gain some voluntary control. Initially, exercises focus on learning to "turn-on" a muscle and then "turn-off" that same muscle.

UPPER EXTREMITY: ARM AND HAND

In Stage Three, the survivor begins to gain some control over the shoulder and elbow. They learn to "shrug the shoulder" bringing it up toward the ear while sitting and then "turn-off" that effort allowing the shoulder to relax. Often, there is a lot of extraneous movement of the neck when learning to shrug the shoulder. That is O.K. Remember, the shoulder region of the cortex is near the neck region so there is some overflow in the instruction pathway. When the survivor is lying on their back, they may also begin to have some control over the shoulder, by bringing both arms up together and then releasing the affected arm, trying to not allow it to fall rapidly back to the bed/mat.

Some control over elbow flexion also begins to develop as the survivor learns to bend their elbow and then "turn-off" the effort and allow the elbow to straighten ~OR~ learn to straighten the elbow and then "turn-off" the effort to allow the elbow to bend. At this stage, we cannot expect voluntary movement between bending and straightening the elbow. It is a matter of actively moving in one direction and then relaxing as gravity or another person helps you into the next. For example, while sitting, an attempt to bend the elbow generally results in partial elbow flexion, accompanied by the shoulder blade pulling back and the hand being dragged over the front of the body. This is a good start. Once accomplished, "turn-off" the effort to bend the elbow, then lean forward allowing gravity to straighten the elbow.

During Stage Three the hand is generally in a fisted position and efforts to exercise will often increase the tone in the hand. It is very important during this stage of recovery to maintain a healthy hand with good range of motion at the wrist and fingers. Daily stretching / massage of the hand is recommended and often a resting splint is needed to keep the hand open during sleeping hours. Specific therapy for the hand is often not successful until the shoulder and elbow have the strength to move the hand toward its target. Remember, a baby begins exploring his environment by bringing a fisted hand toward his mouth or swatting at a toy with a fisted hand. It is not until there is better coordination of the shoulder and elbow that the baby begins to open the hand to interact with his environment.

LOWER EXTREMITY: LEG, ANKLE AND FOOT

During Stage Three, voluntary movement begins to evolve at the hip and knee, but generally not yet at the ankle. The survivor begins to be more able to move the leg while in bed or lying on their back. But, during walking the leg often begins to feel stiffer and very difficult to bend at the knee. Often, stroke survivors become worried that they are getting worse. It is actually just the opposite. The muscles are being driven by a network of brainstem pathways that are providing excitatory signals to the muscles that help to keep the individual upright against the forces of gravity. These brainstem pathways are just not being well modulated by the higher brain that has suffered the stroke. Walking is often limited by this muscle tone and survivors compensate by learning a stiff legged gait with circumduction at the hip. This is complicated by the use of a stiff ankle brace; hence it is necessary to build some ankle motion into an ankle brace at this stage of recovery.

The nervous system has multiple pathways that excite the muscles of the legs during standing, so exercises focused on standing endurance, balance, and stability greatly help strengthen the leg. The key is to learn control over flexion and extension by repeatedly performing a voluntary task. One of my favorite exercises involves learning to move from sitting <-to-> standing independently without the use of the arms to push or pull ones self to standing. Initially this can be practiced from a higher surface and gradually decreasing surface height. It is very important that the ankle not be rigidly constrained by a brace, hence allowing the knee to advance forward over the foot during the sitting <-to-> standing. Once standing, it is important to challenge balance by standing with eyes open, eyes closed, and with very gentle head turn. During standing, sensory signals from the foot help to again activate the muscles of the ankle. Of course, safety comes first so one should always have supervision.

Gait training becomes increasingly important at this stage of recovery and it is imperative that any ankle brace allow dorsiflexion at the ankle. Dorsiflexion is the motion that allows the knee to move forward over the foot during weight bearing, and allows the foot to pull upward to clear the toes when not weight-bearing. Without ankle dorsiflexion, the survivor is doomed to walking with a stiff-legged style of gait with hip-hike and circumduction.

STAGE FOUR:

Synergy patterns still dominant, *but* some movements begin to deviate from synergy. Spasticity begins to decrease. This is an exciting stage of recovery because as the tone is decreasing, voluntary movement begins to evolve out of the fixed patterns of movement often seen in Stage Three.

UPPER EXTREMITY: ARM AND HAND

In Stage Four there begins to be more control of the shoulder and elbow. There is some control over grip with all of the fingers closing simultaneously in a gross grip pattern. The hand generally cannot be voluntarily opened yet, but one can learn to "turn-off" the tension and allow the grip to relax.

Movement combinations of the arm begin to develop. Movements are most easily done while lying supine (on the back). The survivor may be able to straighten the elbow and, using shoulder strength, bring the arm up and over the head. Often the hand will close when the elbow is being straightened, but then the hand will relax once overhead.

While sitting, the survivor begins to be able to bring the hand from lap to chin and also from lap to alternate knee. This requires that the elbow alternate between voluntarily controlled flexion and extension. At this stage, there may also start to be some rotation of the forearm and exercises should focus on alternating between palm-up when the elbow bends to palm-down when the elbow straightens.

While standing, the survivor begins to bring the arm forward with a straight elbow. This is an ideal time to start working on some eye-hand coordination. While standing, one can straighten the elbow and then reach forward toward a tabletop or door. It is also good to gently introduce a moving target such as a soft ball that can be pushed with the hand. The ball can be on a table top, or even gently tossed or rolled by another person.

The hand generally is not opening voluntarily yet, but the survivor can learn to release the tension in the muscles and relax the grip. This is most easily done when leaning forward, since it changes the excitation of the brainstem pathways. For example, one can practice reaching to the floor to pick up a piece of clothing or baby toy, then standing up tall to place the item in the other hand. The forward bend also is useful in lifting a laundry basket with two hands, opening and closing a folding chair with two hands. The general rule I promote during this stage of recovery is that the arm and hand should be used to push, pull, lift and carry.

LOWER EXTREMITY: LEG, ANKLE AND FOOT

The leg tends to progress more quickly through Stage Four than does the arm. However, similar to the hand, the ankle is typically not yet under voluntary control. Recovery of the leg during this stage suggests that the higher brain is now modulating the brainstem pathways. During this stage, the survivor begins to gain more control over the hip and knee.

One may gain control over the ability to flex the hip and knee while lying on their back. A good exercise is to bend the hip and knee such that the foot is planted on the bed/floor and then try to lift the hips off the

74

bed/floor. This exercise – known as bridging – requires coordination between the abdominal muscles, the pelvic and hip muscles, and the muscles of the knee. At first, this may been very disorganized and difficult to perform, but with practice, the many parts begin to coordinate together.

The hip and knee also begin to bend a bit during walking, and the hip is in general much more stable. During walking, the survivor often begins to be able to place the affected foot more midline and carry weight over the leg so that steps become equal in length. Sometimes during this stage, we will see weak activation of the ankle during walking, especially as related to push-off. However, the ability to voluntarily dorsiflex (bring ankle and toes up) is very limited and much too slow for walking. There are a variety of dynamic, tools that can be employed at this stage of recovery. We will discuss these tools more in Chapter Eleven.

STAGE FIVE:

If progress continues, more complex movement combinations are learned as the basic synergies lose their dominance over motor acts. Further decrease in spasticity with relative independence from movement synergies. Tone becomes very low. This is a very rewarding stage of recovery.

UPPER EXTREMITY: ARM AND HAND

In Stage Five there begins to be control of the shoulder in many planes of movement and the elbow can freely move between flexion and extension. The wrist also moves between flexion and extension and there is some control over rotation as well. Strength training and dedicated use of the arm becomes increasingly important in this stage. The tone of the hand decreases. The thumb often moves into an open extended position when the task requires it to do so and the fingers move into a partial extension. Individual finger movement is generally not possible at this stage of recovery but the hand does begin to spontaneously respond to doing tasks. It is important to appreciate that control of the human hand is really task and vision dependent. Most often, our hand is driven by our vision and our desire to accomplish a task. Exercising the hand should incorporate performing a task or a series of tasks. The hand has moved past the stage of push, pull, lift and carry so it can now be employed to grasp, release, turn, twist, tie, etc. I frequently remind clients to observe the skills of a young child as they learn to play using their hands, and develop exercise plans around similar activities.

Lower Extremity: Leg, Ankle and Foot

Control of the leg, ankle and foot continue to evolve in Stage Five. There begins to be control of the hip in many planes of movement and the knee can freely move between flexion and extension. The knee and hip are stable and respond to changes and challenges in the environment. It becomes easier to navigate stairs, curbs and uneven ground. One may have voluntary control of ankle dorsiflexion and plantarflexion during this stage, but the control is usually too slow to be of much use during walking. Often a lightweight ankle brace is all that is required. Electrical stimulation (presented in Chapter Eleven) is also quite successful to assist with the ankle control. Treadmill training is very useful in promoting a faster speed of walking since the survivor is no longer dependent on their arms or external support for balance on the treadmill.

STAGE SIX:

Individual joint movements become possible and coordination approaches normal. There is a continued decrease of spasticity.

This is the goal of recovery, but I personally prefer not to use the word "normal". What is that really? Often one will assume that this means that movement has recovered to the pre-stroke level of energy, strength and coordination. This is not always the case. More often, movement "appears normal". The individual is capable of all daily functional use of the limbs. The arm and hand move freely with individual movement of the fingers returning. Walking is stable and requires no assistive devices. An observer may not be aware of any abnormal movement. However, to the survivor, there may still be some slight reminders/residuals - Often only evidenced during extreme fatigue or stress. It may take more effort to move, especially when fatigued. The fingers and toes may get stiff and slow when cold. The ankle may respond too slowly to run or jump. Movement continues to be difficult with more rapid complex alternating movements, but this too gradually improves with time.

Countless stroke survivors have experienced this continuum of improvement as they meet each challenge with resilience and determination. Each journey to recovery follows a path of highs, lows, and plateaus and with anything human, there is variation and uniqueness.

~ I would rather attempt to do something great and fail than attempt to do nothing and succeed.~

Robert H. Schuller

NOTES:

CHAPTER TEN

REQUIREMENTS FOR LEARNING AND PLASTICITY

In order to move past a plateau, the exercises, lessons and tools must change. Imagine a child attending school and having all of the same lessons in first through twelfth grade. This doesn't make sense with regards to school, so it should not make sense with regards to sensory and motor recovery post-stroke.

The requirements are the same for any learning, and they work for the healthy nervous system as well as an injured nervous system!

1. **ACTIVE PARTICIPATION** – if someone has had an injury to the nervous system, it is not enough that his or her family or loved one wants them to get better. The survivor themselves must engage in getting better. Sometimes that is really difficult. Sometimes people do not actively participate because they can't. They may be depressed, or too exhausted. They may have too many worries about the finances, worrying that they can no longer provide for their family. There are other people whose participation is limited by the severity of their brain injury. The injury may have

affected the brain in such a way that they simply cannot engage. They cannot initiate or take action toward their own recovery. This is very frustrating for their loved ones. *WHY DON'T YOU TRY HARDER? YOU JUST NEED TO DO MORE EXERCISE. YOU NEVER DO ANYTHING IF I DON'T MAKE YOU...* It is important to recognize which battle to tackle first. Sometimes rehabilitation needs to wait until the family has begun to deal with the finances, or until the depression has been properly addressed, or until cognitive therapy and training has addressed the lack of initiation.

2. **USE OF MULTIPLE SENSORY SYSTEMS** - It is really important that whatever you do for rehabilitation, it must include multiple sensory systems. I like to say, "you have to SEE IT, HEAR IT, FEEL IT!" Tools that allow one to see their own performance, hear their performance, and feel their performance will enhance the ability of the nervous system to learn. The nervous system uses sensory feedback to compare how we are doing to how we want to do. Sometimes, one sensory system is substituted for another. Remember, we briefly talked about that in the section on Sensory Substitution.

3. **FEED-BACK TO FEED-FORWARD** – Feed-back occurs when you bump into a wall before you realize that you should have turned to avoid the wall. Feed-forward is when you see the wall and say to yourself "oh yea, I remember..." so you plan a turn and avoid bumping the wall. The nervous system has moved from a "reactive" to a "predictive" behavior. The point is that we cannot predict the need for a correction, if we have never had to react to a mistake. This is sometimes difficult for caregivers because they want to protect their loved one from mistakes.

I remember a gentleman, S.B., who would come into the clinic flanked by his mom. She opened the door for him and guided him through the door ever so carefully. I told her to stop helping him so much and she replied that he needed help so he did not run into the door. Well, the next day, he did run into the door because he had a neglect of his left side. But, what was totally cool is that he only did that a few times before he learned to move over a little bit to avoid bumping into the door.

That is feed-back to feed-forward and that is a subtle sign of improvement and plasticity. One needs to make a lot of mistakes before you can learn.

4. **PRACTICE NEEDS TO BE REWARDING AND IMPORTANT** – how many people feel a lot of personal value and reward from doing 10 repetitions of an exercise. *"1,2,3,4,5,6,7,8,9,10. Good. Now we are done. See you next week."* This does not constitute a therapy session that has been very rewarding or important. But if those 10 repetitions of an exercise had been referenced to how that exercise is going to help you be able to walk again... then it is important. I would caution anyone that if you come home from therapy and your friend or family says "what did you do today in therapy?" and your reply is... "I don't know" then you probably need to speak with your therapist and identify why you are to do that exercise, why you are to spend your insurance dollars on that exercise, what is the benefit of that exercise? If an exercise program is not deemed rewarding and important then you are less likely to practice daily. Less practice leads toward the formidable plateau.

5. **CONSISTENT PRACTICE AND PERFORMANCE** – It is not enough to have a good exercise program. You actually need to have consistent practice. Imagine that you are learning to play the piano. It is not enough to practice only on Monday because your lesson is on Tuesday. In order to really learn, you must practice every day in preparation for your performance at the Tuesday lesson. As a therapist, it is so rewarding to send someone away with an exercise program/a plan for recovery and when they come for their next session they have improved! That is learning. And learning means that the nervous system is changing. That is neuroplasticity.

6. **REPETITION, REPETITION, AND THEN SOME MORE REPETITION** – I suppose this goes along with consistent practice, but the requirement for repetition is important. Some *variability* needs to be built into repetition. It is not enough to perform repetitions of a single movement. Motor learning requires interaction with the environment. During gait training, I tell my clients that their goal is to reach 1000 steps per day. Perhaps initially, they can only walk 22 steps and require more than one minute to walk a distance of 10 feet. Well, at least that is a starting point. Their exercise program incorporates daily standing and daily walking. Improvement is noted when someone can walk the same distance with less assistance, walk the same distance in less time, OR a walk a greater distance in the same time.

These requirements for neuroplasticity have led me toward an interest in using more tools during therapy and a lot less instruction or hands-on treatment. It seems that with the appropriate tool, there is a guarantee that the six above mentioned requirements are met. A combination of direct hands-on assisted exercise with a home program that utilizes tools to assist repetitive exercise may promote more rapid and long-term recovery.

In the following chapter, I will be introducing various tools that are currently available for rehabilitation, but for now let's just consider the use of a treadmill for gait training.

Most patients that are beginning to regain their ability to walk can walk on a treadmill. Having a body-weight support system or an overhead harness is helpful but not critical. Having someone physically available to help and keep the patient safe is critical. A gait belt must be worn, and the treadmill must have an emergency stop tether. It is NEVER advised to try walking on a treadmill without a trained professional first assessing your ability and safety.

Given that the assessment has been completed, and safety is assured then the treadmill is a tool that can be employed to meet the requirements for neuroplasticity. A 2008 review publication (Forrester, Wheaton, Luft) provides evidence that treadmill training can contribute to neuroplasticity in survivors recovering from stroke. The brain actually changes as a result of the exercise.

1. *ACTIVE PARTICIPATION*– the moving belt establishes a requirement to actively participate and move the feet. Generally, stroke survivors can begin treadmill training at a speed of 0.5 or 0.6 miles per hour.

2. *USE OF MULTIPLE SENSORY SYSTEMS* – *"see it"* - speed, distance walked, time walked, etc. are displayed on the control panel *"hear it"* – the sound of the

belt moving, the sound of the feet striking *"feel it"* - the legs moving, the feet striking the belt, the amount of weight support.

3. ***FEED-BACK TO FEED-FORWARD*** – initially stepping in response to the belt movement is a feedback response. The belt moves and therefore the feet must react. Sometimes physical assistance is required to help move the feet in a reciprocal stepping pattern. However, as one continues to walk on the treadmill, this reaction begins to train the nervous system for anticipation. As a therapist, I know a patient is beginning to use anticipatory control when they can walk faster.

4. ***REWARDING AND IMPORTANT*** – being able to record either more time walked on the treadmill or a faster treadmill speed is rewarding and walking is important. Most of my clients have told me that the ability to walk is one of the most valuable skills they can regain. With walking comes independence, but also humanity.

5. ***CONSISTENT PRACTICE AND PERFORMANCE*** – as with anything in life, practice leads to improved performance. I recommend setting a schedule for exercise – actually blocking it off on your calendar as an appointment with yourself. Walking is therapeutic in so many ways. It frees the mind and strengthens the body.

6. ***REPETITION*** – walking on the treadmill allows for high repetition stepping. Repetition, practice and performance allow the brain to move from feed-back to feed-forward. One of my daughter's

violin instructors had a poster on her wall that said, "Perfect practice makes perfect". I never agreed with this and felt that it was limiting my daughter's practice time. She felt that if she did not play everything perfectly then it was not a good practice session. We changed instructors. She learned to enjoy the practice time and found that each week she improved. It is the repetition, repetition, repetition that forms a pathway in the brain.

Establishing a pathway in the brain is similar to establishing any path or route. I live in the Sierra Foothills, surrounded by the rich history of the Gold Rush. Imagine the difficulties those earlier pioneers must have faced. Each step forward was toward the unknown and through some of the most formidable obstacles. But, once a path was established the route became easier and easier to follow. A simple path through the rough terrain became a paved freeway. So is it with the nervous system. The more it is used, the stronger and faster a simple connection becomes.

~ As a single footstep will not make a path on the earth,
so a single thought will not make a pathway in the mind.
To make a deep physical path, we walk again and again.
To make a deep mental path, we must think over and over
the kind of thoughts we wish to dominate our lives. ~

Henry David Thoreau

NOTES:

CHAPTER ELEVEN

EMERGING TOOLS IN REHABILITATION

There are many routes to recovery. No one perspective or approach to rehabilitation therapy provides everything necessary to the survivor. Listed in alphabetical order, each has its own merits. I would encourage you to learn more about these techniques and how they may apply to an individual stage of recovery. Whichever approach is chosen should match the needs of the individual recovering from neurological injury. More often than not, recovery requires much time and money so it is prudent to understand why a particular approach is being taken before allocating your resources. Remember also that many senior centers, YMCAs, and community colleges also provide opportunities to work with personal trainers and participate in group-exercise classes.

~ ACUPUNCTURE ~

~ ALEXANDER TECHNIQUE ~

~ CONSTRAINT INDUCED MOVEMENT THERAPY (CIMT) ~

~ BIOFEEDBACK THERAPY ~

~ BoTox Injections ~

~ Dardinski Method ~

~ Feldenkrais Method ~

~ Kawahira Method ~

~ Neuro Developmental Treatment (NDT) ~

~ Neuro-Ifrah ~

~ Proprioceptive Neuromuscular Facilitation (PNF) ~

~ Pilates ~

~ Weight Training ~

~ Yoga ~

Many therapists and trainers use a combination of approaches, often in combination with some of the emerging tools in rehabilitation. Just as neuroscience research has exploded, so has the development of tools that – at least in theory – apply current knowledge of neuroplasticity to the rehabilitation of an injured nervous system. I want to stress that these tools do not replace the need nor the importance of physical and occupational therapy. In fact, I think that these tools supplement therapy and allow the therapy to have an even stronger impact on recovery. These tools are not meant to replace stretching, strengthening, and balance training, but rather to augment these. Most insurance will allow PT/OT for a fixed number of visits each year with a new prescription. Your therapist may have learned of a new tool in the time since your last therapy appointment.

Not every tool is the right tool for each survivor, but at

the very least rehabilitation therapists, survivors and their families should be aware of what is available in neurological rehabilitation. Included in this chapter are the tools that I have had the opportunity to employ in my clinical practice as well as some that are soon to be released. This list is by no means inclusive of all the rehab products available and there is not yet substantial research into the effectiveness of these tools.

It is important to note that inclusion of these tools and discussion of their application does NOT – either directly or indirectly - infer an endorsement of the tools or companies. Any omissions from this list are not intentional.

It is the responsibility of the reader and their own rehabilitation team to determine which, if any, of these tools may be helpful in their own rehabilitation. I believe that with introduction of the appropriate tools, rehabilitation professionals can better promote ongoing recovery from stroke and other neurological injuries. The tools can often be implemented into a home exercise program and may help the motivated survivor meet the requirements for learning and neuroplasticity.

If you are interested in learning more about any of the tools listed, I would encourage you to contact the companies directly and ask to speak with one of their representatives. It is likely that a local rehab or gym facility in your area has one or more of these tools. The list is organized alphabetically with their websites and United States phone numbers provided.

UPPER EXTREMITY RECOVERY & HAND REHABILITATION:

ARMEO®
http://www.hocoma.com
USA Phone: 781-792-0102

~

BIONESS H200 WIRELESS HAND REHABILITATION SYSTEM
http://www.bioness.com
USA Phone: 800-211-9136

~

BIOXTREME'S REHABILITATION ROBOTICS SYSTEM - DEXTREME™
http://bio-xtreme.com
USA Phone: 877-486-5998

~

INTERACTIVE MOTION TECHNOLOGIES
http://interactive-motion.com
USA Phone: 617-926-4800

~

MEDÍTOUCH – HAND TUTOR
http://www.meditouch.co.il/HandTutor
USA Phone: 512-608-8638

~

MYOMO
http://www.myomo.com
USA Phone: 877-736-9666

~

SAEBO
http://www.saebo.com
USA Phone: 888-284-5433

~

LOWER EXTREMITY RECOVERY & GAIT REHABILITATION:

ALTERG – ANTIGRAVITY TREADMILL® AND ALTERG BIONIC LEG®
http://www.alterg.com
USA Phone: 510-270-5369

~

BIONESS L300 FOR FOOT DROP
http://www.bioness.com
USA Phone: 800-211-9136

~

BLUEROCKER™ OR TOEOFF®
http://www.allardusa.com/
USA Phone: 888-678-6548

~

DYNAPRO ELITE AFO
http://www.pattersonmedical.com
USA Phone: 800-343-9742

~

EKSOBIONICS - Ekso™
http://www.eksobionics.com
Multiple sites in USA

~

KICKSTART
http://www.cadencebiomedical.com
USA Phone: 877-484-7513

~

LITEGAIT
http://www.litegait.com
USA Phone: 800-332-9255

~

LOKOMAT®
http://www.hocoma.com
USA Phone: 781-792-0102

~

REWALK
http://www.rewalk.com
USA Phone: 877-799-9255

~

SOLO-STEP
http://www.solostep.com
USA Phone: 866-631-1117

~

WALK-AIDE
http://www.walkaide.com
USA Phone: 888-884-6462

~

SPEECH RECOVERY

Although I do not have expertise in speech recovery, I do want to mention that there are many assistive devices and training aides to help with speech rehabilitation. Many of the same principles of neuroplasticity apply to speech recovery. I would encourage readers to learn more about the wealth of resources and technologies.

National Aphasia Association
http://www.aphasia.org
USA Phone: 800-922-4622
e-mail: naa@aphasia.org

Anecdotally, some past clients have also found that foreign language software has been helpful in their ability to regain spoken language. Instead of trying to access a lost language, they "learn" a new language. For example, if the ability to speak English has been lost, then the foreign language they learn is English.

Rosetta Stone®
http://www.rosettastone.com
USA Phone: 800-767-3882

COGNITIVE RECOVERY

There are a number of different types of software programs and books to help recover functions related to memory, attention, problem solving and mathematics. Listed in alphabetical order are those that I have employed. This list is by no means inclusive of all products available and any omissions from this list are not intentional.

Brain Training Games by Lumosity
http://www.lumosity.com
submit request via website for more info

BrainHQ from Posit Science
http://www.positscience.com
submit request via website for more info

Low-tech brain exercises may include many of our favorite games:

Battleship

Blokus

Boggle

Card games

Checkers

Coloring books

Jenga

Hidden word puzzles

Scrabble

Tetras

Please remember that at first, the stroke survivor may require assistance with any tool or exercise. Recovery is a daunting task. Socialization and encouragement during any activity helps to provide motivation. Respect provides dignity.

~ *Exercise the muscles* ~ *Exercise the brain.*~

CHAPTER TWELVE

SIMPLE RULES TO PROMOTE IMPROVEMENT
~ Not listed in any specific order ~

- Have Hope.
- Have Patience.
- Celebrate success.
- Seek resources and ask for help.
- Move past the "Plateaus" on your journey.
- Keep your mind open to changing perspectives.
- Accept your injury as "the reason" not "your excuse".
- Surround yourself with people who believe in you.
- Set reasonable goals. Once reached, set new ones.
- Discover what you can do and then do more of that.
- Demand more of your health care professionals.
- Learn from your past. Don't try to regain it.
- Use your senses: "See it, hear it, feel it".
- Change your tools as you change.
- Notice small improvements.
- Vary the task demands.
- Learn from mistakes.
- Participate in life.
- Learn to Laugh.
- Show Love.

NOTES:

Appendix

References and Recommended Reading

References

Bach-y-Rita P. "Brain Plasticity" In: *Rehabilitation Medicine*. edited by J. Goodgold, 113-118. Mosby Inc. 1988.

Bach-y-Rita P and Kercel SW. "Sensory substitution and the human–machine interface". *TRENDS in Cognitive Sciences* 7, Dec (2003): 541-546.

Begley S. *Train your mind change your brain: How a new science reveals our extraordinary potential to transform ourselves.* Ballantine Books a division of Random House, Inc, New York: NY, 2007.

Blakemore C. "Achievements and challenges in The Decade of the Brain." *EuroBrain* 2, March (2000): 1-4.

Bobath B. *Adult hemiplegia: Evaluation and treatment.* London: Spottiswood Ballintype, 1978.

Brunnstrom S. "Motor testing procedures in hemiplegia: based on sequential recovery stages." *Physical Therapy* 46 (1966): 357–375.

Brunnstrom S. *Movement therapy in hemiplegia: A*

neurophysiological approach. Medical Dept. Harper & Row, New York: NY 1970.

Cajal, S Ramón y. *Estudios sobre la degeneración y regeneración del sistema nervioso*. Moya, Madrid, 1913.

Cajal, S Ramón y. "Degeneration and regeneration of the nervous system." In *History of Neuroscience*, edited by DeFelipe J, Jones EG, Translated by May RM. Oxford University Press, Inc. 1991.

Caramia MD, Iani C, Bernardi G. "Cerebral plasticity after stroke as revealed by ipsilateral responses to magnetic stimulation." *Neuro Report* 7 (1996): 1756-1760.

Carr JH, Shepherd RB, Nordholm L, and Lynne D. "Investigation of a new motor assessment scale for stroke patients." *Physical Therapy* 65 (1985): 175–180.

Cao Y, Vikingstad EM, George KP, Johnson AF and Welch KMA. "Cortical language activation in stroke patients recovering from aphasia with functional MRI." *Stroke* 30 (1999): 2331-2340.

Chollet F, DiPiero V, Wise RJS, et al. "The functional anatomy of motor recovery after stroke in humans: A study with positron emission topography." *Annals of Neurology* 29 (1991): 63-71.

Colucci-D'Amato L, Bonavita V, and Di Porzio U. "The end of the central dogma of neurobiology: stem cells and neurogenesis in adult CNS." *Neurological Neuroscience* 27:4 (2006): 266-270.

Cramer SC, Nelles G, Benson RR, et al. "A functional MRI study of subjects recovered from hemiparetic stroke." *Stroke* 28 (1997): 2518-2527.

Cramer SC. "Repairing the human brain after stroke: I. Mechanisms of a spontaneous recovery." *Annals of Neurology* 63 (2008): 272-287.

Danilov YP, Tyler ME, Skinner KL and Hogle RA. "Efficacy of electrotactile vestibular substitution in patients with peripheral and central vestibular loss." *Journal of Vestibular Research: Equilibrium & Orientation* 17, no. 2,3, (2007): 119-130.

Doidge N. *The brain that changes itself: stories of personal triumph from the frontiers of brain science.* Viking – Penguin Group, New York: NY 2007.

Forrester LW, Wheaton LA, Luft AR. Exercise-mediated locomotor recovery and lower-limb neuroplasticity after stroke. *Journal of Rehabilitation Research & Development* 45, no. 2 (2008): 205-220.

Grafman J and Litvan I. "Evidence of four forms of neuroplasticity." In *Neuronal Plasticity: Building a bridge from the laboratory to the clinic: research and perspectives in neurosciences,* Springer Berlin Heidelberg, 1999: 131-139.

Hachisuka K, Umezu Y and Ogata H. "Disuse muscle atrophy of lower limbs in hemiplegic patients." *Archives of Physical Medicine & Rehabilitation* 78 no. 1 (1997): 13–18.

Hafer-Macko CE, Ryan AS, Ivey FM and Macko RF. "Skeletal muscle changes after hemiparetic stroke and potential beneficial effects of exercise intervention strategies." *Journal of Rehabilitation Research & Development* 45, No. 2 (2008): 261–272.

Hallet M. "Plasticity of the human motor cortex and recovery from stroke." *Brain Research and Reviews* 36 (2001): 169-174.

Herculano-Houzel, S. "The human brain in numbers: A linearly scaled-up primate brain." *Frontiers in Human Neuroscience* 3, no. 31 (2009): 1-11.

Holloway V, Gadian DG, Vargha-Khadem F, et al. "The reorganization of sensorimotor function in children after hemispherectomy. A functional MRI and somatosensory evoked potential study." *Brain* 123, no.12 (2000): 2432-2444.

Hosp JA and Luft AR. "Cortical plasticity during motor learning and recovery after ischemic stroke." *Neural Plasticity* (2011).

James W. "The principles of psychology" (1890). In The *principles of psychology volume I and II*. Harvard University Press, 1981.

Jauch EC, Caver JL, Adams HP, et al. "Guidelines for early management of patients with acute ischemic stroke: A guideline for health care professionals from the American Heart Association/ American Stroke Association." *Stroke* Mar (2013): 1-78.

Kaas JH. "Neuroanatomy is needed to define the "organs" of the brain." *Cortex: a journal devoted to the study of the nervous system and behavior* 40, no. 1 (2004): 207-208.

Krakauer JW. "Arm function after stroke: From physiology to recovery." Seminars in *Neurology* 25, no. 4 (2005): 384-395.

Kübler-Ross E. *On Death and Dying*. Scribner, New York: NY 1969.

Kübler-Ross E and Kessler D. *On Grief and Grieving*. Scribner, New York: NY 2005.

Liepert J, Miltner H, Bauder H, et al. "Motor cortex plasticity during constraint-induced movement therapy in stroke patients." *Neuroscience Letters* 250 (1998): 5-8.

Luft AR, Forrester L, Macko RF, et al. "Brain activation of lower extremity movement in chronically impaired stroke survivors." *Neuroimage* 26, no.1 (2005): 184-194.

Macko RF, DeSouza CA, Tretter LD, et al. "Treadmill aerobic exercise training reduces the energy expenditure and cardiovascular demands of hemiparetic gait in chronic stroke patients: A preliminary report." *Stroke* 28, no. 2 (1997): 326–330.

Macko RF, Ivey FM, Forrester LW, et al. "Treadmill exercise rehabilitation improves ambulatory function and cardiovascular fitness in patients with chronic stroke: A randomized, controlled trial." *Stroke* 36, no.10 (2005): 2206-2211.

Murphy TH and Corbett D. "Plasticity during stroke recovery: from synapse to behavior." *Nature Reviews Neuroscience* 10, Dec (2009): 861-872

Ouellette MM, LeBrasseur NK, Bean JF, et al. "High-intensity resistance training improves muscle strength, self-reported function, and disability in long-term stroke survivors." *Stroke* 35, no. 6 (2004): 1404–1409.

Poliak S, Peles E. "The local differentiation of myelinated axons at Nodes of Ranvier." *Nature Reviews Neuroscience* 4, Dec (2003): 968-980

Potempa K, Lopez M, Braun LT, et al. "Physiological outcomes of aerobic exercise training in hemiparetic stroke patients." *Stroke* 26, no. 1 (1995): 101–105.

Roland PE, Larsen B, Lassen NA, Skinhoj E. "Supplementary motor area and other cortical areas in organization of voluntary movements in man." *Journal of Neurophysiology* 43 (1980): 118-136.

Ryan AS, Dobrovolny CL, Smith GV, et al. "Hemiparetic muscle atrophy and increased intramuscular fat in stroke patients." *Archives of Physical Medicine and Rehabilitation* 83, no.12 (2002): 1703–1707.

Sampaio E, Maris S, Bach-y-Rita P. "Brain plasticity: 'visual' acuity of blind persons via the tongue." *Brain Research* 908, no. 2 (2001): 204-207.

Sawaki L, Butler AJ, Leng X, et al. "Constraint-Induced Movement Therapy results in increased motor map area in subjects 3 to 9 months after stroke." *Neurorehabilitation Neural Repair* 22, Sep-Oct (2008): 505–513.

Sawner KA and LaVigne JM. *Brunnstrom's movement therapy in hemiplegia: A neurophysiological approach*, 2nd ed. Philadelphia: J.B. Lippincott, 1992.

Schwartz JM and Begley S. *The mind and the brain: Neuroplasticity and the power of mental force.* Harper Collins Publishers, Inc. New York: NY 2002.

Smith GV, Forrester LW, Silver KH, Macko RF. "Effects of treadmill training on translational balance perturbation responses in chronic hemiparetic stroke patients." *Journal of Stroke and Cerebrovascular Disease* 9, no.5 (2000): 238–245.

Smith GV, Macko RF, Silver KH, Goldberg AP. "Treadmill aerobic exercise improves quadriceps strength in patients with chronic hemiparesis following stroke: A preliminary report." *Neurorehabilitation and Neural Repair* 12, no. 3 (1998): 111–118.

Twitchell TE. "The restoration of motor function following hemiplegia in man." *Brain* 74 (1951): 443–480.

Winstein CJ, Marians AS, Sullivan KJ. "Motor learning after unilateral brain damage." *Neuropsychologia*, 37 (1999): 975-987.

Yang YR, Wang RY, Lin KH, et al. "Task-oriented progressive resistance strength training improves muscle strength and functional performance in individuals with stroke." *Clinical Rehabilitation* 20, no.10 (2006): 860–870.

About the Author:

Anne Burleigh Jacobs, PT, PhD earned her physical therapy degree from the University of Colorado in 1985 and a doctorate in Neuroscience and Physiology from the Oregon Health Sciences University in 1995. Dr. Jacobs' research and clinical interests over the past 25 years have focused on the role of sensory and motor interactions for recovery of standing balance, ambulation, and reaching movements post neurological injury. Dr. Jacobs was a co-founder of the Peninsula Stroke Association (now Pacific Stroke Association) a non-profit organization dedicated to stroke prevention, support and advocacy. Currently, she specializes in post-stroke recovery through her private practice, provides research consultation to technology companies and teaches neuroscience and movement science courses in a variety of forums. Dr. Jacobs was a contributor to the textbook Neuroscience: Fundamentals for Rehabilitation, and she has lectured nationally and internationally on topics related to neuroscience, recovery of sensory-motor function, and motor learning.

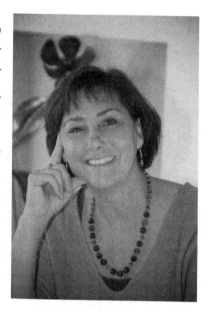

Photograph by Julie Shaw

Made in the USA
San Bernardino, CA
10 July 2015